Is Gluten Free 4 You?

Is Gluten Free 4 You?

Why you should – and why you shouldn't –

consider going gluten free: the astonishing

evidence

Marie Pendle-Clarke

Dedication

To Nick

Disclaimer

The information contained in this book is not intended to give dietary advice and is not a substitute for medical guidance and treatment from a suitably qualified health professional. If the information contained in this book raises questions or concerns about your health, you are advised to consult with your GP or physician.

Table of Contents

Introduction

ecent years have seen a huge rise in the popularity of the gluten free diet, with the gluten
ee global food market revenues estimated at 2.4 billion dollars in 2014 and predicted to
se to 4.8 billion dollars by the end of 2021 (Transparency Market Research, 2018).
he gluten free diet, which requires the exclusion of the three primary grains of wheat,
arley and rye from a person's diet, has historically been solely associated with coeliac
isease and dermatitis herpetiformis. Coeliac disease is defined by the World
astroenterology Organisation as '*a chronic, multiple-organ autoimmune disease that affects
he small intestine in genetically predisposed children and adults. It is precipitated by the
ngestion of gluten-containing foods.*' (World Gastroenterology Organisation, nd). This
utoimmune disorder affects about 1% of the population worldwide, whereby the ingestion
f gluten causes damage to the small intestine, resulting in malabsorption of vital nutrients.
he lifelong adoption of a strict gluten free diet is recognised globally as the only known
reatment for coeliac disease to date.

owever, millions of people worldwide who do not have a diagnosis of coeliac disease are
onsuming gluten free foods. Indeed, such is the popularity of the diet that people with a
nedical diagnosis constitute only a small percentage of those consuming gluten free foods
lobally. It is the vast number of non coeliacs apparently driving the demand and market for
luten free products. It appears that there are many more reasons why people are choosing
o consume these products. Some perceive it to help with weight loss; others see it as a
ealthier option. Many people report a reduction in abdominal discomfort, bloating and pain
hrough the adoption of the gluten free diet and some with conditions such as Irritable
Bowel Syndrome report benefits from the diet.

But is a gluten free diet helpful or harmful to people? Maintaining good health means making
nformed choices. For some, a gluten free diet is not a lifestyle choice, but a medically

recommended treatment and the only way to stay well. For many others, the marketing messages and headline statements made about gluten, wheat and other grains can be confusing and misleading. How do we know what and who to believe as we strive for good health?

What exactly is gluten and why is it the latest pariah? How easy is it to follow a gluten free diet and can we be sure that what we are eating is genuinely gluten free? Is the gluten free diet truly a panacea for many ills or is it actually harmful to health?

This book examines some of the research behind the hype. It aims, in a clear, straightforward way, to guide the reader through the myriad scientific studies attempting a answer to these and many more questions.

Following such a restricted diet should only be undertaken under medical supervision. It is hoped that the information in this book can help to inform the conversation with your medical practitioner.

Background

I am not a scientist, medical doctor, nutritionist or dietician. I do have a Doctorate in Education and experience of reviewing academic literature, studies, claims and assertions. I have also been on a gluten free diet for nearly 40 years, since I was diagnosed with coeliac disease in 1980.

The recent growth in popularity of the diet I find really intriguing. I wanted to explore the reasons behind its apparent popularity and why people who do not have coeliac disease would choose to follow such a restrictive regime. Approaching this task as a lay person attempting to make sense of all of the information out there, my research led me to believe that there are many so-called 'facts' surrounding the diet that both coeliacs and non coeliacs need to know about, in order to make informed choices and to be able to live a healthy life. It is not for me to say what people should or should not believe. I do not wish to add to the confusion with sweeping, unfounded statements or claims. I have not conducted my own research in this area and am not qualified to do so. I have, however, attempted to provide the reader with information on what rigorous scientific research tells us about gluten and wheat, and given some pointers for assessing the credibility of the competing media claims, to help to make sense of what we are being told. It may not provide all the answers you need but, to excuse the pun, will hopefully give you 'food for thought'.

My story

My journey with gluten began at the age of fifteen, when, for some reason, I started being ill. I like to think I can pinpoint the exact moment my healthy, happy teenaged body turned against me, although to date, I still don't have a satisfactory explanation for why I suddenly had an adverse reaction to gluten. I recall sitting in French class and my intimidating teacher creeping up behind me and slamming his fists on the desk because I couldn't answer a question he had asked. I nearly jumped out of my skin. I guess I would have thought no more about the incident, except that the very next day my whole body had blown up: my lips, face, arms and legs swollen into a rash of huge hives. I looked – and felt – hideous. The doctor could only see me in a week's time and by the time I was seen, the rash was barely visible. It - and I – was dismissed. I then began a slow decline, losing weight, vomiting, becoming anaemic; being told at first that it was exam nerves, then probable anorexia, and then maybe leukaemia. My parents were beside themselves. I was being seen regularly for iron injections and examined monthly by a paediatric consultant (paid for privately by my grandfather), but eventually I became so weak that I couldn't walk and I was eventually admitted to hospital. I weighed barely 80 pounds (under six stone) and needed an urgent blood transfusion. I was told later it was touch and go whether I would make it. A couple of days later, a gentle doctor asked if my parents were on any medication and when I told him about my father's Dapsone tablets for his skin condition (dermatitis herpetiformis), an urgent biopsy was ordered and I finally had a diagnosis – coeliac disease. By this time I was nearly eighteen years old.

I was immediately put on a gluten free diet and I could only feel utter relief that the problem was finally solved. Within weeks, I began to gain weight. My appetite was almost insatiable and I observed with joy the colour of my nails turning pink again. I didn't have a problem with the diet. It was working and I was beginning to regain my strength and my health. I was advised that there was a lot of damage to my small intestine and that some damage may be irreparable, but I was a happy teenager again, and I accepted unconditionally that I would never be able to have gluten again, even in the smallest amounts.

The fast food culture in 1980 was just taking off. I had never eaten a pizza, had a McDonald's or even been out for many restaurant meals. My favourite food to eat at home was chips, eggs, beans and bacon and I would have readily eaten this three times a day, had I been allowed. I began to love the taste of food again and would pile up my plate, enjoying every single mouthful. I rarely had any cravings for disallowed food. My biggest problem was embarrassment and social awkwardness at mealtimes. I was different. I had this strange disease that no-one understood and I couldn't join in with my peers. Although I was at that awkward teenage period anyway, I can confidently say that I have felt this exclusion keenly for a good part of my gluten free life. One of my earliest awkward moments was having to refuse some peanuts being offered to me by a college guy I had a crush on, because they were coated in flavourings. He thought I wasn't interested in him and that was the end of that. In the early years, it was not uncommon for my meal to be served last in any restaurant. Often I had to send something back because of a lack of understanding of what a gluten free meal meant. I regularly waited whilst others tucked in, and then ate alone whilst their plates were being whisked away. I have had to refuse invitations out when the restaurant menu wasn't suitable and refuse invitations to dinner when I didn't want to explain about my strange diet or submit my hosts to the burden of catering gluten free, particularly in the early years when gluten free alternatives were not readily available. I have never wanted to draw attention to myself, yet being on a gluten free diet does precisely that. I have been to functions and events and had a discreet word about my dietary requirements, only to find, with the best of intentions, a huge plate, wrapped in film with my name on it, highlighted as if painted neon with flashing lights, prompting embarrassing questions and discussions about my bodily functions at mealtimes. At work, whilst they endeavoured to cater for me in the best way they could, I have often had to balance a plate of salad or a baked potato on my knee, along with a knife and fork, whilst the rest of the team have sandwiches, walk around and mingle. The mild embarrassment and social exclusion have probably been the biggest negatives of the diet for me. I have, therefore, in many ways embraced the rise in popularity of the gluten free culture. I no longer have to launch into long, rambling explanations or give up and choose a salad. I love seeing gluten free menus in restaurants or being given the option to tick gluten free on catering requests. Supermarket shopping has become exciting again.

However, this explosion in awareness and availability has not been without its problems for me. I was filling my cupboards with lovely treats – croissants and cakes and crumpets and quiche. I was delighting in the choice and taste of a sliced loaf, a bread roll, a pitta and a wrap. I could have a ready-made sandwich, a sausage roll, a pizza or a pie. I was gaining weight. I went out for my first gluten free pizza at a regular restaurant chain and was thrilled. I was severely ill the next day and for weeks afterwards. I was eating delicious biscuits and crackers labelled gluten free but not feeling good. I was struggling to stay well. Doing the research for this book I have discovered some of the reasons why this may be the case. It has been a revelation.

There is no question that if you have coeliac disease, dermatitis herpetiformis or gluten ataxia, then the only way to stay healthy is to follow a strict gluten free diet. Gluten free is without doubt for you. However, a gluten free diet is not without its issues and controversies.

This book highlights some of the current scientific research on the gluten free diet and its effects and what the clever marketing industry fails to reveal to the unsuspecting consumer. The evidence is truly astounding.

Chapter 1 outlines exactly what gluten is, just to clear up any misunderstandings about this protein, and identifies the main reasons why a significant percentage of the global population is currently so keen to avoid it. In Chapter 2, the medical conditions for which a gluten free diet is the only treatment are discussed, along with the problems in maintaining a strict gluten free diet, such as labelling, lack of agreement on the definition of gluten free and issues of cross contamination. The perception that a gluten free diet is healthier and promotes well being is addressed in Chapter 3, looking at the evidence from robust scientific investigations on nutrition, heart health, diabetes and sports performance. The evidence veals much that we, as consumers, are not being told! Chapter 4 assesses the belief that a

uten free diet can help with weight loss. The scientific evidence on gluten and obesity is

uly shocking. The phenomenon of gluten sensitivity is discussed in Chapter 5, and whether

umans are actually evolved to tolerate gluten. Current scientific research in this area is

evealing some surprising results that we may well be backing the wrong horse with gluten!

nally, in Chapter 6, the weight of evidence against gluten and grains is considered, with

ompelling research on the function and effect of grains on our bodies. This is scientific

formation we ignore at our peril.

hope that the information and research evidence contained in this book allows for a more

formed debate on the relative merits of a gluten free diet and I sincerely hope that the

urrent food industry enthusiasm for gluten free continues - but not at the expense of the

ealth and wellbeing of us as consumers.

xx

Definitions of scientific terms

Anecdotal evidence: data that usually comprises people's personal experiences. The evidence cannot be said to apply to the wider population, it cannot be checked independently and there are no controls for other factors that may be at play.

Blind study: a study where researchers and/or participants are not aware of which study group they are in, so that they cannot inadvertently influence the results.

Single blind study: Participants do not know whether they are in the experimental group or the placebo group.

Double blind study: Neither researchers nor participants know which group they are in.

Cross-over study: A study design that compares 2 or more interventions. For example, group 1will be given intervention A followed by intervention B. Group 2 will be given intervention B followed by intervention A. Effects are compared on participants, rather than between participants.

Literature review: A summary and conclusion of findings from range of published studies.

Meta-analysis: A review of the results of several studies investigating the same question, where the data is combined and analysed to assess the overall impact of the intervention. Results are considered more accurate and reliable when several studies are taken into account, rather than relying on the results of one study. Systematic reviews may use meta-analysis.

Placebo: A fake pill or treatment with no effects. It cannot be distinguished from the real pill or treatment. The aim is to establish the impact of the real treatment and control for the possible psychological effects of being given treatment.

Prospective cohort study: A study with 2 or more cohorts (groups) of participants who share similar characteristics. One group has a treatment or symptom or has a particular risk factor. The other group does not. The participants are observed over a length of time and their progress monitored.

Prospective study: A study, usually over a long period of time, which monitors outcomes (such as a disease or condition) during the study period. The outcomes are examined for links to suspected risk factors or protective factors.

Retrospective study: A study which examines past exposure to suspected risk factors or protective factors for a particular outcome (such as a disease or condition).

Systematic review: Systematic methods are used to identify, select and evaluate studies relevant to a particular research question. Findings from the studies are collated and analysed, sometimes using statistical techniques such as meta-analysis. Again, as several studies are analysed, the findings are considered more accurate and reliable.

Chapter 1

Gluten, grains, aches and pains

What is gluten?

Gluten is a storage protein or prolamin, found in certain cereals. Cereals are also known as grains.

Cereals derive from the grass family and produce edible, starchy seeds that are harvested for food. Examples of these cereals include rice, maize, wheat, barley, rye, oats, sorghum, quinoa and millet. Some of these cereals contain gluten and some do not.

Cereals, including gluten-containing cereals, contain vitamins, minerals, protein, fats, oil and carbohydrates required for human health.

> The cereals of **wheat, rye and barley** and their derivatives all contain gluten.

In **wheat**, the storage protein is a combination of predominantly two proteins called gliadin and glutenin.

In **barley**, the storage protein is hordein.

In **rye**, the storage protein is secalin.

Together, these prolamins are commonly referred to as **gluten**. Thus, wheat, barley and rye all contain gluten.

Oats contain a different protein, called **avenin**, which is similar to gluten. Whether oats contain gluten is a separate debate discussed in Chapter 2.

The word gluten derives from the Latin name for glue and the late 16th century French word for 'sticky substance'. The gluten protein creates the elasticity in certain foods, including bread. Because of its properties, it is often added to processed foods to enhance the taste, texture and moisture content (Biesiekierski, 2017).

Contain gluten

Wheat	Bulgur wheat	Durum wheat
Barley	Pearl Barley	Semolina
Couscous	Spelt	Triticale
Einkorn	Rye	Kamut
Malt	Emmer	Freekeh

Whole grains versus processed grains

Whole grains are the entire seed. In the field, all grains are in this natural whole grain state, with the seed covered by a protective, inedible husk. Whole grains are comprised of bran, endosperm and germ, which are all edible.

Bran contains omega 3 fatty acids, fibre, vitamins and minerals.

Endosperm contains mainly carbohydrates and proteins.

Germ contains vitamin E, folate, thiamine, phosphorus and magnesium.

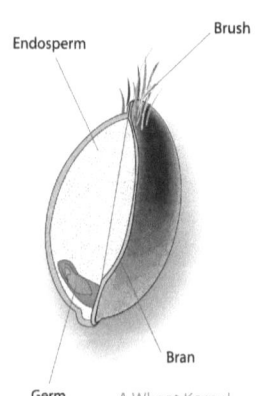

A Wheat Kernel

Adapted from Phu Thinh Co Wheat-kernel_nutrition

https://www.flickr.com/photos/phuthinhco/7610266772

Cereals are considered to be staple food crops, with wheat being the predominant crop. These staple food crops provide more food energy worldwide than any other type of crop with many billions of people in various parts of the world relying particularly upon rice, wheat and maize daily for their survival (Sarwar, et al, 2013). It is estimated that over 50% of the world's calorie intake is derived from these crops (ibid).

Why are we eating so much wheat?

In Britain during the Second World War the Nutrition Society was formed, whose remit was to actively encourage and promote global crop production with high nutritional value, within the context of rationing and concerns about the health and nutrition of the peoples of countries at war (Copping, 1978). By the end of the 20th Century, wheat production had increased five-fold (Aziz et al, 2015).

Amongst all the grains, wheat is now one of the most globally traded and consumed food crops (Biesiekierski, 2017). Wheat contains proteins, B vitamins, fibre and minerals. It can be grown in large quantities and produce quality yields. In particular, however, it is the gluten in the wheat that makes it ideal for bread making, providing the glutinous structure of the dough. Gluten is also added to many processed foods to improve taste and texture (Biesiekierski, 2017). Currently, about 95% of all wheat grown is bread wheat, which is a hybrid of emmer (a cultivated ancient wheat grain) and wild grass (Brouns, et al, 2013, Aziz, et al, 2015). Durum wheat comprises the bulk of the rest of the wheat crop, with small amounts of other forms of wheat such as einkorn and spelt being grown (Brouns, et al, 2013).

Wheat contains between 8-15% protein and of this protein, around 90% comprises gluten (Biesiekierski, 2017).

In the Western world, it is calculated that we are consuming an average of between 10-15g of gluten per day (ibid).

> Gluten provides the elasticity in dough, its properties making it excellent for bread making. It is also added to processed foods to improve taste and texture.

The gluten free revolution

The avoidance of gluten in a diet has historically been associated with people with a diagnosis of coeliac disease. Coeliac disease is a genetic, autoimmune disorder, whereby the ingestion of gluten causes an inflammatory response in the intestine, damaging the lining, leading to malabsorption of essential nutrients. This, in turn, leads to a range of health complications, including anaemia, fatigue, and osteoporosis. To date, the only known treatment for coeliac disease is to follow a strict, gluten free diet.

The incidence of coeliac disease worldwide is considered to be around 1% of the population (Lerner et al, 2015), although in recent years it has been noted that the prevalence of coeliac disease appears to be on the rise globally (White et al, 2013, Lerner et al, 2015, Offord, 2017). The reason for this is still unclear. It may be a result of increased awareness and diagnosis of coeliac disease, with a simple blood test now routinely used to screen for particular antibodies (Shewry and Hey, 2016). However, some have suggested that the rise in incidence is linked to the rise in the production and consumption of grains such as wheat (Aziz et al, 2013). There is some evidence that changes in technology relating to the production of wheat have increased exposure to gluten (Biesiekierski, 2017). Nevertheless, coeliac disease remains relatively uncommon, yet the gluten free food industry has seen a rapid growth in recent years, with this explosion in awareness, production and availability of gluten free products way out of proportion to the rise in the incidence of coeliac disease (Reilly, 2016).

So, to what can this thriving market in gluten free products be attributed?

Gluten is currently being charged with causing many disorders, including heart disease, diabetes and obesity. There is a popular perception that it is bad for you, and is being treated as a pariah in our modern diet. Thus, we are witnessing an increasing trend towards the avoidance of gluten.

Data on health and wellness trends from Euromonitor show that the largest growth area from 2012 -2017 was the gluten free market, with the US, the UK and Italy predominantly driving this growth (Mascaraque, 2018).

Prominent media discourses - celebrities and bloggers, high profile athletes and the popular press -have fuelled the dissent about gluten with an estimated 20% of Americans (The Hartman Group, 2015), 12% of Australians (Hendrie et al, 2016) and 22% of people in the UK (Mintel, 2016) avoiding wheat/gluten.

Several surveys have been undertaken to identify reasons for people adopting this gluten free diet.

A Mintel Report in 2014 revealed that it is non coeliacs who are driving the gluten free food market, citing some remarkable statistics (Topper, 2014). The survey revealed that:

- Only 18% of those who eat or have eaten gluten free foods do so because of a diagnosis of coeliac disease.

5

- Of the 82% who eat gluten free without a diagnosis, just over half of them do so due to self diagnosed gluten intolerance or sensitivity.
- 38% of people eat, or have eaten gluten free food due to perceived health benefits of the diet.
- A quarter of the consumers surveyed gave weight loss as a reason for eating gluten free foods.

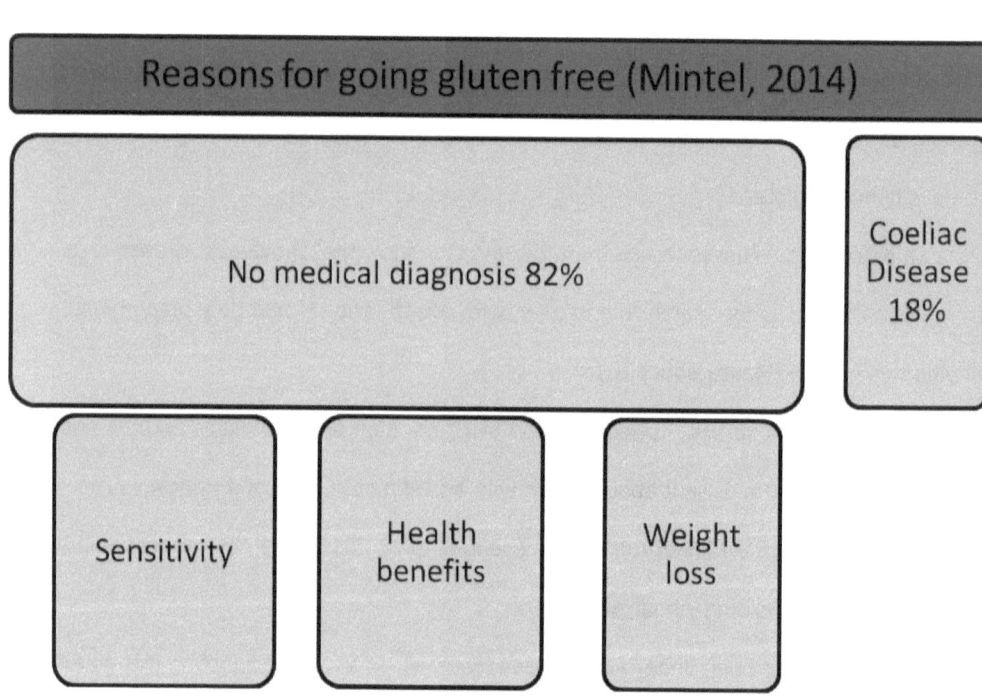

Similarly, a Hartman Group survey in 2015 highlighted the following reasons:

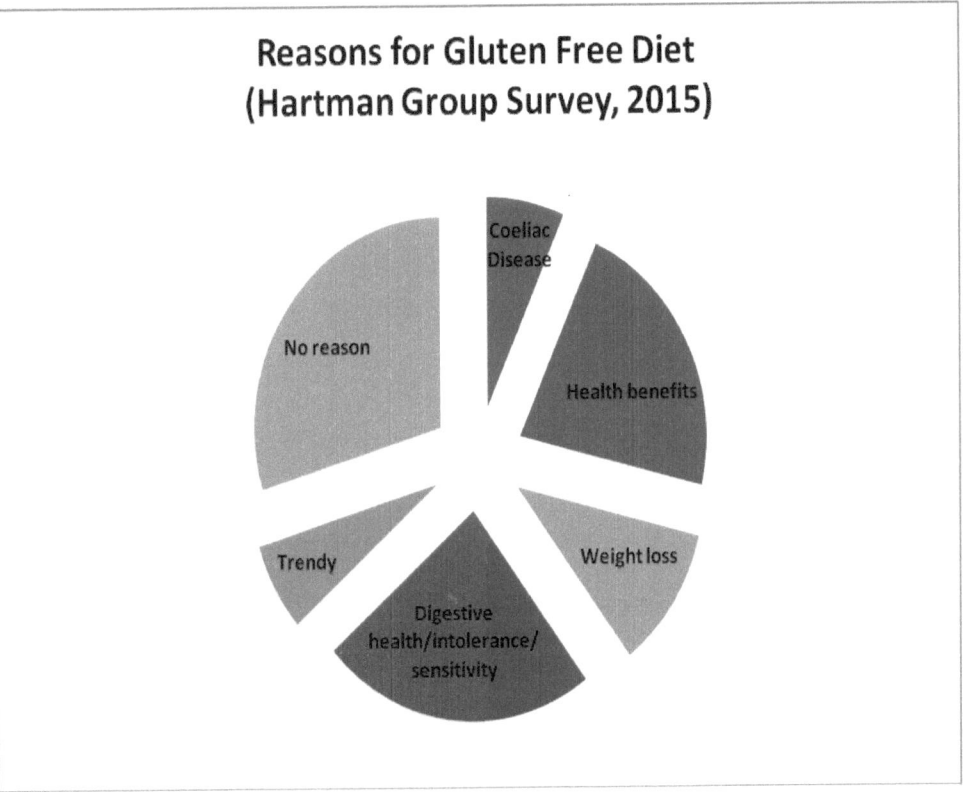

There are different reasons why people adopt a gluten free diet, with coeliac disease being one of the least common reasons. A major factor appears to be the association of a gluten free diet with improved health.

A DuPont Nutrition and Health survey (Hamann, 2017) reported that the perceived health benefits of gluten free items are the main motivation for initial purchasing of these products and that the 'gluten free' claim is the most important health claim on food labels for consumers. The main health benefits are considered to be:

- Improves digestive health

- Helps with weight loss

- Improves overall health and wellbeing

The survey reports that this perception of gluten free being a healthier alternative is being driven by the media, with non coeliac bloggers, celebrities and athletes promoting its benefits.

Gluten and wheat are certainly being blamed for a host of ailments and diseases, from digestive problems to cardiovascular disease and diabetes (Davis, 2011). Is it any wonder that the global gluten free food market has seen rapid growth? According to a report by Global Market Insights, the market was worth just under 4 billion dollars in 2013 (Adams, 2017) and estimated at just under 15 billion dollars in 2016 (Grand View Research, 2017). In summary, there appear to be four main reasons why people adopt a gluten free diet, apart from having no reason, or seeing the diet as trendy. Following the diet on medical advice due to a diagnosed condition is the least cited reason. Many are self diagnosing as being sensitive to gluten and avoiding gluten to reduce gastrointestinal symptoms. Others just perceive a gluten free diet to contribute to their overall health. Some report following the diet in an effort to lose weight.

The vast majority of people are following a gluten free diet without medical advice or supervision, convinced of the benefits through information provided by the popular press, social media, celebrities, word of mouth and advertising. But is a gluten free diet really helpful for people without a medical diagnosis? Can we rely upon blogs, celebrity endorsements and anecdotal reports for our health and wellbeing, or should we be looking to science and robust empirical evidence to inform our dietary choices?
What is the evidence about the benefits of a gluten free diet?

4 main reasons for adopting a gluten free diet

Diagnosed medical condition

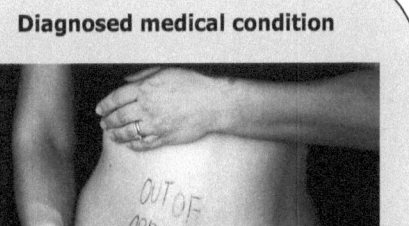

Health benefits

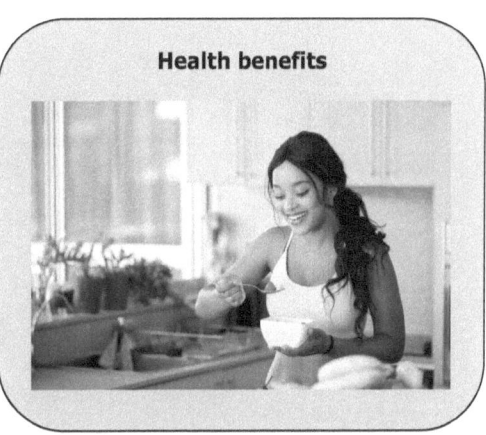

Weight loss

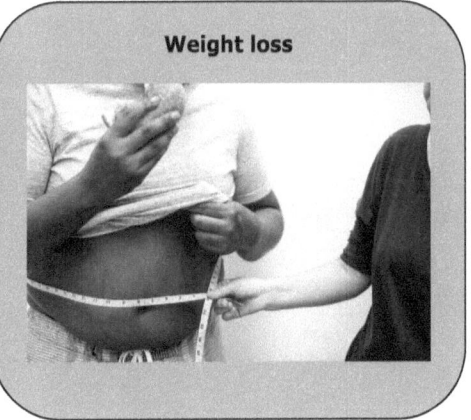

Self diagnosed sensitivity

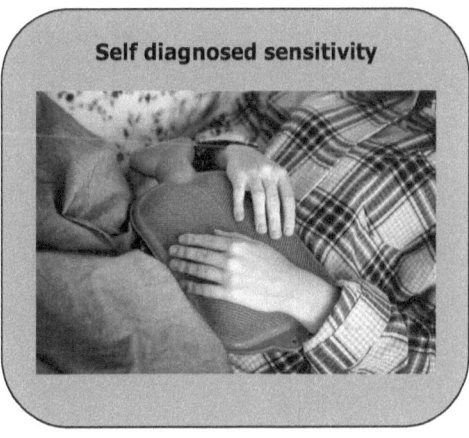

Marie Pendle-Clarke

Chapter 2

When gluten free is the only way to be

Diagnosed Medical Conditions

For people with coeliac disease, dermatitis herpetiformis and gluten ataxia, lifelong adherence to a strict gluten free diet is the medically recommended advice for the remission of symptoms and for the maintenance of good health. A gluten free diet is the globally accepted treatment for these autoimmune conditions.

Due to the intestinal damage that even small amount of gluten can cause with these conditions, it is vitally important to stay vigilant with food, read food labels carefully and ensure that, as far as is possible, the ingestion of gluten is totally avoided. Whilst going gluten free appears a simple remedy for these autoimmune disorders, it is a challenging diet and not without its controversies.

Did you know...?

- Just a crumb of gluten can be harmful to coeliacs?
- Gluten free oats may not necessarily be safe for coeliacs?
- Some naturally gluten free foods may be contaminated?
- Eating gluten free in a restaurant is not guaranteed to be safe for coeliacs?

The importance of strict adherence to the diet cannot be underestimated, by those having to follow the diet and those catering for people with these autoimmune conditions. Gluten is very harmful. The avoidance of gluten is paramount. It is not a lifestyle choice.

Coeliac Disease

Coeliac disease is an autoimmune condition whereby the ingestion of gluten causes inflammation and damage to parts of the small intestine. The small intestine is where the nutrients from food get absorbed into the bloodstream through the villi – millions of tiny hair like structures than line the small intestine, increasing its surface area. In people with coeliac disease, gluten causes an adverse reaction in the gut, creating inflammation and causing the villi to be shortened or completely flattened, thus restricting the surface area and causing malabsorption of nutrients.

There is a genetic predisposition to coeliac disease. This is marked by the carrying of the human leukocyte antigen (HLA) DQ2 or DQ8 (Biesiekierski, 2017).

Symptoms

Symptoms can vary widely amongst people with coeliac disease, which often makes it difficult for the medical profession to quickly recognise the condition. It is known to be under-diagnosed (Aziz, 2015) and mis-diagnosed (El Salhy et al, 2015).

Typical symptoms include:

> Anaemia

> Fatigue

> Vomiting

> Nausea

> Weight loss

> Diarrhoea

➢ Headaches

➢ Bloating

➢ Stomach pains and cramps

Untreated, it can lead to other complications such as fertility problems and osteoporosis. It has been noted (Aziz et al, 2015) that the classic symptoms of coeliac disease – diarrhoea, failure to thrive and anaemia, are less evident in patients nowadays than they were fifty years ago. More commonly, patients present with Irritable Bowel Syndrome type symptoms, iron deficiency, osteoporosis and ataxia (ibid). This may, in part, contribute to the under diagnosis and mis-diagnosis of the condition.

Diagnosis

Diagnosis of coeliac disease can be a two- step process. Undiagnosed coeliacs produce antibodies in the bloodstream as a reaction to the gluten. A simple blood test can be used to screen patients, which can detect whether these antibodies are present in the blood. However, a definitive diagnosis can only be given by checking for damage to the villi in the small intestine. Therefore, the blood test is normally followed by a jejunal biopsy, where a small sample of the intestine is taken for microscopic inspection. If someone suspects that they may have coeliac disease, it is advised that they do not embark on a gluten free diet before diagnosis, as it is then much more difficult to detect the damage to the intestine. Thus there is less confidence in the diagnosis.

Treatment

Coeliac disease is successfully treated through the adoption of a strict, gluten free diet. This treatment is recognised worldwide as the only effective solution to the amelioration of the symptoms experienced, and to the repair of the villi in the small intestine.

A Dutch paediatrician called Willem-Karel Dicke is attributed with the discovery of the gluten free diet as a treatment for coeliac disease. He identified wheat as the culprit causing the coeliac symptoms and experimented with wheat free diets, publishing his first report on the benefits of this diet to coeliacs in 1941 (van Berge-Henegouwen and Mulder, 1993).

Dermatitis Herpetiformis

Dermatitis herpetiformis is a chronic autoimmune skin condition that is associated with coeliac disease. It is caused by a reaction to the ingestion of gluten.

Symptoms

 Dermatitis herpetiformis is characterised by an itchy, blister like rash, predominantly on the elbows, knees and buttocks, although it can appear on other parts of the body. The rash is usually symmetrical, for example appearing on both elbows or both knees. Many people with dermatitis herpetiformis do not report the gut symptoms of people with coeliac disease, but damage to the villi in the small intestine is often present.

Diagnosis

Diagnosis of dermatitis herpetiformis is initially through a skin biopsy to check for a particular antibody. If this antibody is present, then the next step is a test for coeliac disease through blood tests and jejunal biopsy.

Treatment

The treatment for dermatitis herpetiformis is lifelong adherence to a gluten free diet. In addition, tablets (dapsone) may initially be prescribed to help alleviate the skin rash symptoms. (Coeliac UK, nd)

Gluten Ataxia

Gluten ataxia is a relatively new and still not a fully recognised condition (Fletcher, 2018). It is classified as an autoimmune disorder, whereby ingestion of gluten affects the cerebellum - a part of the brain (Sapone et al, 2012). This causes neurological difficulties with movement.

Symptoms

Gluten ataxia affects balance, leading to lack of coordination, clumsiness and slurred speech as a result of a reaction to the ingestion of gluten. Neurological symptoms can present in people with coeliac disease but they can also be present on their own. Damage to the gut will not necessarily be seen in everyone with gluten ataxia, although it is estimated that around a third of patients will present with damage (Sapone et al, 2012).

Diagnosis

Currently, the advice to medical professionals is to screen for particular antibodies. If these antibodies are elevated, an intestinal biopsy would be performed to check for damage to the intestine. Since intestinal atrophy will not be seen in all patients with gluten ataxia, it is advised that patients presenting with these antibodies put on a strict gluten free diet. Improvement of symptoms after 12 months on the diet would strongly support a diagnosis of gluten ataxia (Sapone et al, 2012)

Treatment

Treatment is a strict, lifelong gluten free diet (Coeliac UK, nd). It is advised that patients are monitored to check for the elimination of the antibodies after 6 to 12 months on the diet (Sapone et al, 2012).

Wheat allergy

Wheat allergy is not the same as gluten intolerance or coeliac disease. Wheat allergy is a histamine response to the wheat grain, where the immune system reacts abnormally to contact with wheat.

Symptoms

Wheat allergy causes symptoms such as itching, swelling, rash and asthma. It can also cause wheezing and anaphylaxis which is life threatening (Mulder et al, 2013).

Diagnosis

Wheat allergy can be detected through a simple allergy test.

Treatment

Treatment includes strict avoidance of wheat. As gluten is a protein in wheat, then this usually means that gluten is avoided too. However, it is not the gluten protein that causes the allergic reaction. It is the wheat grain. Symptoms can be alleviated with antihistamines and corticosteroids and epinephrine in case of anaphylaxis (Mulder et al, 2013).

The difference between a wheat allergy and coeliac disease

There is often much confusion around wheat allergy and coeliac disease, but they are two distinct, different conditions.

Coeliac disease is not an allergy to gluten. It does not cause the typical allergic (histamine) response. Accidental ingestion of gluten in coeliac disease does not generally cause an immediate response, although occasionally some people can experience immediate symptoms of vomiting and abdominal pain. It causes inflammation in the gut, when it passes through the intestines.

A wheat allergy does not cause the intestinal damage seen with the autoimmune response to gluten in coeliacs. Instead, it causes many typical allergic symptoms. People will generally be aware within minutes to hours that they have come into contact with wheat (Sapone et al, 2012).

The incidence of wheat allergy is around 0.4% of the world's population (Biesiekierski, 2017), which is rarer than the estimated 1% of the population affected by coeliac disease. The three medical conditions of coeliac disease, dermatitis herpetiformis and gluten ataxia are an immunological response to gluten in the small intestine causing observable inflammation and damage to the absorption surface in the intestine. To avoid ingesting gluten, one must avoid the three grains of wheat, barley and rye and their derivatives.

In contrast, wheat allergy is an immediate allergic response just to the wheat grain. Avoiding wheat is advised, but other grains including barley and rye do not cause an allergic reaction and can therefore be consumed. Thus, a wheat free diet is less restrictive than a gluten free diet.

Gluten free is not necessarily wheat free!

Some gluten free products are manufactured from wheat with the gluten part extracted. These products are not suitable for someone with a wheat allergy. Ingredients need to be checked carefully to see if they contain gluten free wheat starch.

Wheat free is not necessarily gluten free!

Products can be advertised as wheat free. These products are suitable for someone with a wheat allergy. However, some wheat free products can contain barley or rye. These products are not suitable for coeliacs, as barley and rye contain gluten. Merely eliminating wheat does not therefore eliminate gluten from the diet.

Gluten free is NOT the same as wheat free
Wheat free is NOT the same as gluten free

Is gluten free food actually free of gluten?

Despite worldwide acceptance that a gluten free diet is the 'gold standard' treatment for coeliac disease, aspects of the diet are still problematic for coeliacs. These include:

- The definition of gluten free
- The case for oats in the diet
- Issues of cross contamination
- Eating out

Defining gluten free

Did you know...?

The same product can be deemed safe for coeliacs to eat if you are in the US, but unsafe for coeliacs to eat if you are in New Zealand?

There is no globally accepted definition of what it means for a food to be gluten free. There is an international body called Codex Alimentarius that is responsible for setting standards for food. The Codex standard states that only foods that contain no more than 20 parts per million (ppm) of gluten, can be labelled as gluten free. This is equivalent to 20 grams per kilogram. A product containing no more than 100ppm may be labelled as 'low gluten'.

Many countries have decided to adopt this as their standard for gluten free foods, including the UK and Europe. In the EU, legislation since 2012 states that food can only be labelled as gluten free if it contains less than 20ppm.

In the United States, the Food and Drug Administration (FDA), whilst not adopting the Codex standard, has developed its own standard, which is the same as Codex Alimentarius in that a food must contain less than 20ppm to be labelled gluten free. This is voluntary guidance and not subject to strict enforcement.

In Australia and New Zealand, the national standard for a food to be labelled gluten free is less than 5ppm. Thus, the same product can be deemed safe for coeliacs to eat in the USA and unsafe to eat in New Zealand!

Why the disagreement about what is deemed to be gluten free?

The US FDA argues that it is currently not possible to detect gluten at levels lower than 20ppm with available analytical methods (FDA, 2017), which is one of the reasons it adopted this threshold. Yet, in New Zealand it is claimed that test kits can detect as low as 3ppm (Coeliac New Zealand, nd). The FDA also argues that there is evidence that most coeliacs can tolerate very small amounts of gluten with no damage to the intestine. Therefore, there is no necessity for a 'zero gluten' approach to food testing and labelling (FDA, 2017). However, the safe level of consumption of gluten in coeliacs can vary, with estimates of between 10 – 100mg day (Biesiekierski, 2017). Coeliacs are also warned of the dangers of even small crumbs having the potential to be damaging, and are advised to avoid cross contamination (Coeliac UK, nd). Due to the wide variation in tolerance to gluten in the coeliac population, there is little consensus on the threshold of gluten that should be set – the level that is safe for coeliacs to consume.

Of course, vested interests are also at stake here. As testing methods become more sensitive, food manufacturers are concerned that foods will no longer meet the gluten free criteria (Biesiekierski, 2017). Thus, how we define what is meant by gluten free remains controversial (Mulder, et al, 2013). It is certainly a fine balance between encouraging manufacturers to enter the gluten free market and provide more choice and variety in gluten free foods, and ensuring that the health and wellbeing of coeliacs is protected.

Country	Definition of gluten free
Europe	Less than 20ppm
UK	Less than 20ppm
US	Less than 20ppm
Canada	Less than 20ppm
New Zealand	Less than 5ppm
Australia	Less than 5ppm

In conclusion, many foods labelled gluten free actually do contain gluten, albeit small amounts – less than 20 parts per million (20 milligrams of gluten per kilogram of food).

Is there a safe level of gluten consumption for coeliacs?

In 2016 a systematic review of 18 studies was undertaken to try to establish a safe level of gluten consumption in coeliacs (Reid et al, 2016). It concluded that there was moderate evidence that consumption of 50mg gluten per day caused intestinal damage. However, the effects of consuming between 2 and 10mg gluten per day were difficult to establish in the studies. The researchers stated that there is a wide variance in individual tolerance to gluten, making it difficult to establish a safe threshold of gluten consumption.

With the current explosion of alternative gluten free products on the market, coeliacs may be exposing themselves to more gluten than previously. Where coeliacs may have had an apple as a snack, a gluten free muffin can now be enjoyed, or a packet of gluten free pretzels. Very small amounts of gluten are being consumed each time. Is it possible that even this 20ppm threshold could be harmful to some coeliacs? How much gluten free food might it take to invoke a reaction in sensitive coeliacs?

20ppm equates to 20 milligrams (mg) of gluten per kilogram of food, or 10mg per 500 grams (g) of food.

Thus, consuming 500g of gluten free food at 20ppm in one day would lead to ingestion of 10mg gluten. Consuming this amount of gluten free food would be very difficult to do if following the recommendations for a healthy, balanced diet. However, it is not impossible to consume 500g gluten free food in one day.

The general advice in the UK is that coeliacs can safely consume unlimited amounts of gluten free products containing 20ppm or less as this very small amount has not been shown to be toxic (Coeliac UK, nd). Furthermore, as 20ppm is the upper threshold, many products test at far lower than this, to allow for a margin of error.

Nevertheless, maintaining a balanced diet is very important. In addition, given the current paucity of evidence on safe levels of gluten consumption, it is worth considering whether having a bagel for breakfast, perhaps a mid morning muffin, sandwiches for lunch, a few cookies, then pasta or pizza for dinner and cake for dessert, with all products containing some gluten (albeit less than 20ppm), is prudent, no matter how tempting.

> **Many products labelled gluten free do contain gluten, albeit it in very small amounts, ranging from less than 3 mg per kilo up to 20 mg per kilo.**

Naturally gluten free foods

There are foods that naturally do not contain gluten. These include fresh meat, fish, potatoes, vegetables, fruit, eggs, dairy products, nuts and seeds.

There are also a range of naturally gluten free grains and flours, and these have become more widely available in recent years, through supermarkets and health food stores.

Naturally gluten free grains/flours

Corn or Maize	Rice	Buckwheat
Teff	Millet	Polenta
Quinoa	Hemp	Sorghum
Tapioca	Sago	Flax
Gram/chickpea	Urid	Chestnut
Arrowroot	Potato	Coconut

Are naturally gluten free grains and flours safe for coeliacs?

Just because these grains and flours are naturally gluten free doesn't mean that they are automatically safe for coeliacs to eat. Agricultural practices of crop rotation, transport, milling and storage give rise to opportunities for gluten free grains to come into contact with gluten-containing grains, leading to a chance of cross contamination. It is not always clear on the packaging whether this is the case, as naturally gluten free products will not necessarily have a gluten free label. It is assumed that products with a gluten free label will have been rigorously tested to ensure compliance with the national standard.

However, studies have found that contamination can and does occur in both naturally gluten free products and those labelled gluten free.

A study in Canada (Koerner et al, 2013) analysed 640 naturally gluten free products used by coeliacs, that were sold in shops and through the Internet between 2010 and 2012. The researchers found that

- Nearly 10% of these products contained more gluten than the recommended 20mg per kilogram (20ppm).
- The highest level of contamination showed nearly 8,000 milligrams per kilogram.
- Over 1% of the products labelled gluten free were tested as being over 20ppm, with the highest gluten content showing 141mg per kilogram.
- Typical foods that were contaminated included soy, millet and buckwheat.

A study in the US (Lee et al, 2014) calculated the gluten content of 78 food samples labelled gluten free, randomly collected from various markets in Idaho.

- 20.5% (16) samples contained more than 20mg per kg, ranging from 20.3 – 60.3mg per kg
- Five out of eight breakfast cereals had a gluten content higher than the recommended 20mg per million.

A study in Italy (Verma et al, 2017) looked at the gluten content of 200 products randomly selected from different supermarkets, that were both naturally gluten free and certified gluten free according to the Codex standard. The study found that:

- 9% of products contained gluten higher than the recommended level of 20ppm – between 20.4ppm and 126.2ppm.
- Those products certified gluten free were less likely to be contaminated by gluten.
- Typical contaminated foods were oats, buckwheat and lentils.

A study in Spain (Bustamante et al, 2017) traced the degree of gluten contamination in 3141 samples of gluten free cereal based products from 1998 to 2016. The researchers detected gluten in 371 samples (almost 12%), concluding that there had been a decline in gluten detection of foodstuffs over time, possibly due to the implementation of the Codex standard and stricter guidelines on food labelling. However, they concluded that whilst foods are now generally safer, flour samples containing over 100mg per kg (100ppm) gluten have risen since 2013, indicating that strict controls need to be maintained.

In 2015, Genius Foods, a leading gluten free manufacturer in the UK, recalled a number of their products due to contamination in a factory they own. Foods marketed as gluten free were shown to contain up to 80ppm of gluten. Whilst considered to be at the 'low gluten' threshold, it was significantly higher than the Codex 20ppm allowed for a gluten free claim. Genius stated that it identified and removed the source of the contamination, whilst conducting additional checks and quality assurance procedures (Coeliac UK, 2015).

People who are required to follow a strict gluten free diet may be understandably disquieted by these studies, as there is a lot of trust placed in the manufacturers of gluten free foods. Contamination can –and does- occur.

When choosing naturally gluten free products, particularly flours, care and vigilance are required. Many companies do adhere to strict standards and is advisable to check with your Coeliac Society group for recommended manufacturers.

It may be argued that gluten contamination cannot be totally avoided (Collin et al, 2004). Nevertheless, it is incumbent on manufacturers who produce and market foods for the gluten free market to remember that whilst the market share of those with coeliac disease and other medical conditions is much smaller than others who are choosing a gluten free diet, gluten contamination can be very dangerous for coeliacs. Strict testing and safety must be paramount, whilst enjoying the boom of the trend.

Are oats gluten free?

In the US, UK and EU, oats are considered to be gluten free if they have been tested to contain less than 20ppm of gluten. Thus, the advice generally given to coeliacs by the medical professionals in these countries is to avoid oats unless they are labelled as 'gluten free' oats. In reality, 'gluten free oats' describe oats have been produced in a gluten free environment, with no risk of contamination. These types of gluten free oats are now widely available, not just as a stand-alone produce, but frequently included in other products such as biscuits, that are labelled gluten free.

However, controversy surrounds the inclusion of oats in the gluten free diet (Biesiekierski, 2017). There appears to be no consensus in the scientific community about the safety or otherwise of oats for coeliacs, and this is reflected in the conflicting advice given in different countries around the world to coeliac patients.

Oats contain the protein avenin. In the literature, avenin is can be variously referred to as a gluten protein (Creed, 2016, Biesiekierski, 2017) or similar to gluten (Coeliac UK, nd, Celiac Disease Foundation, 2014).

In Australia and New Zealand, oats are not considered to be gluten free. Under the Food Standards Australia New Zealand (FSANZ) Food Standards Code, no product that contains oats is allowed to be labelled gluten free, even if tested to contain less than 5ppm of gluten. This is due to evidence that the consumption of oats can cause the same inflammatory response as wheat in some people with coeliac disease (Creed, 2016). The advice on the New Zealand coeliac website is for coeliacs to avoid oats, in addition to the other three grains.

Can 'gluten free' oats be harmful to coeliacs?

Various studies have investigated the effects of oat consumption on people with coeliac disease, with conflicting findings.

A five year Finnish study of 63 patients in 2002 concluded that ingestion of oats does not harm people with coeliac disease (Janatuinen et al, 2002). Thus, the recommendation for coeliacs in Finland is that oats are generally safe in moderate amounts for most people.

A study in 2003 (Lundin et al, 2003) of 19 patients reported findings that villous atrophy had been observed in one patient through the consumption of pure oats (uncontaminated), and concluded that it is highly likely that some patients with CD may be intolerant to pure oats.

A systematic review (Pulido et al, 2009) of the scientific evidence regarding the safety of pure oat consumption in coeliacs concluded that a small number may not be able to tolerate pure oats.

The difficulties in drawing any firm conclusions from such research arise, according to Pulido et al (2009) from various limitations to the studies, including the lack of long-term research into oat ingestion, the small sample sizes of the groups challenged with oats and the lack of detail on the reasons why certain participants withdrew from the studies.

Nevertheless, the research would appear to indicate that there is a small subgroup of coeliac patients unable to tolerate pure, uncontaminated oats (Pulido et al, 2009, Fric et al, 2011).

Avenin comprises just 10-15% of the total protein content of oats, whereas the gluten in wheat is a substantially higher concentration, at 80-85% of total protein content (Gilissen et al, 2016). This lower protein content may, in part, contribute to coeliacs' greater tolerance of oats. Nevertheless, studies on the oat protein avenin have shown not only that it can induce an inflammatory response in some coeliacs, but also that the potential toxicity of oats depends upon the variety (Real et al, 2012). Some cultivars appear to be non-toxic whilst others have been shown to induce inflammation in coeliac patients (Silano et al, 2014). Furthermore, in a study in 2014, analysis of certain pure oats found the presence of gluten at more than the legislated level of 20ppm in three oat varieties (Benoit et al, 2017). This has led researchers to conclude that some oat varieties may well cause problems for some coeliacs (Maglio et al, 2011, Benoit et al, 2017, Silano et al, 2014).

Clearly more research in this area is needed. It has been suggested that it is possible to cultivate varieties of oats that do not induce the inflammatory effect in coeliacs (Giminez et al, 2017).

Brouns et al (2013) also concluded that due to the positive effects of grains on general health, it is important that the food industry looks at developing alternative crops that do not contain gluten, such as oat, teff, quinoa and chia, to assist in the promotion of a healthy diet for coeliacs.

Country	Oat recommendation for coeliacs
United States	Pure oats safe (tested at 20ppm or less)
Europe	Pure oats safe (tested at 20ppm or less)
UK	Pure oats safe (tested at 20ppm or less)
Canada	Pure oats safe (tested at 20ppm or less)
Finland	Pure oats safe (tested at 20ppm or less)
New Zealand	Pure oats not safe
Australia	Pure oats not safe

Currently, coeliacs are advised to seek advice and monitoring from a dietician, with regard to the inclusion of oats in their diet.

Is it safe to eat out gluten free?

It has often been difficult for coeliacs to find gluten free food items away from home. However, the rise in the popularity of the gluten free diet has widened availability of gluten free foods substantially, with many restaurants and eating establishments now offering gluten free menu items and even a separate gluten free menu. In the US, a gluten free menu is available in around 10% of restaurants (Mintel, 2015). Whilst this development may be welcomed, questions remain about whether a food industry keen to attract gluten free consumers is completely aware and committed to the food awareness and standards required to keep customers safe and well who can be severely damaged by gluten.

The regulations that were put in place in 2014 regarding the labelling of foods as gluten free extend to restaurant meals. However, there are issues around staff awareness and the potential for cross contamination, which makes it difficult for the consumer who can become very ill through the ingestion of small amounts of gluten.

A study in the UK (Aziz et al, 2014) sent questionnaires to 265 chefs in Sheffield in 2013, to investigate their awareness of coeliac disease and gluten related disorders. Researchers found that 78% chefs were aware of coeliac disease and almost 88% were aware of gluten related disorders. Certainly, the rise in popularity of the gluten free diet has raised awareness in the catering community. But does this translate into safe practices?

In a recent study in Australia (Halmos, et al, 2018) researchers randomly selected 127 food outlets in Melbourne, Australia that advertised food menu options that were gluten free. Unannounced visits were made and samples of food items taken for analysis. The results indicated that 9% of gluten free food items sampled were not compliant with the definition of gluten free (5ppm) laid down by Food Standards Australia New Zealand (FSANZ) as they contained detectable gluten when tested. Furthermore, 6% of the samples contained more than the Codex standards of 20ppm. Researchers also found that one business provided wheat based items in a meal, containing more than 80ppm. It was concluded that gluten can be found in gluten free foods in restaurants in Melbourne and that more knowledge and training is needed to protect people who depend on a strict gluten free diet for their health.

Whilst it is law that information on allergens are available for all meals served in restaurants (Coeliac UK, nd), unless the restaurant has gluten free accreditation, there is no way of knowing the standard of compliance with regard to food preparation and serving. For example, when gluten containing foods and gluten free foods are being prepared on the same premises, a distance of at least 2 metres is required between preparation areas in order to avoid cross contamination, according to research (Miller, 2016).

It is not enough that the food item itself is gluten free. It is imperative that things like preparation surfaces, toasters, fryers and cooking utensils such as pans, spoons, etc. are kept separate for the preparation of gluten free foods and ideally labelled clearly, so that all staff are aware, in order to avoid cross contamination. Just frying gluten free chips in the same oil as battered onion rings can cause harm to coeliacs.

Clearly, foods and establishments that are certified gluten free offer a greater degree of certainty to coeliacs as testing, awareness raising and standards have been implemented in order to gain accreditation.

As the gluten free industry continues to expand and restaurants continue to profit from this growth in demand for gluten free food items and menus, coeliacs and those whose health critically depends upon a strict gluten free diet should not be forgotten. As consumers, it is important that questions are asked of the restaurants regarding their food safety and compliance, to try to keep healthy and to raise awareness that for some people, this is not a lifestyle choice.

Chapter 3

Can we be healthier and happier when gluten free?

Many people are turning to a gluten free diet due to the perception that going gluten free will have a positive effect upon their health and wellbeing. Some well known celebrities and athletes are among those espousing the benefits of a gluten free diet, many of whom are not diagnosed with coeliac disease, but following the diet for its apparent health appeal. According to a Mintel survey in 2014, nearly 40% of people consuming gluten free foods were doing so not because of a diagnosed medical condition requiring a gluten free diet, but because of the perceived health benefits. Similarly, in a Hartman Group survey in 2015, 26% of those surveyed cited 'healthier option' as the reason for purchasing gluten free foods.

More recently, a DuPont Nutrition and Health consumer survey (2018) also revealed that the European markets for gluten free foods are being driven by non –coeliac consumers' desire for a healthy lifestyle.

Is a gluten free diet scientifically evidenced to be a healthier choice?

Popular belief:

Gluten free foods are more nutritious than their gluten containing counterparts. A gluten free diet therefore has health benefits.

Are gluten free foods healthier?

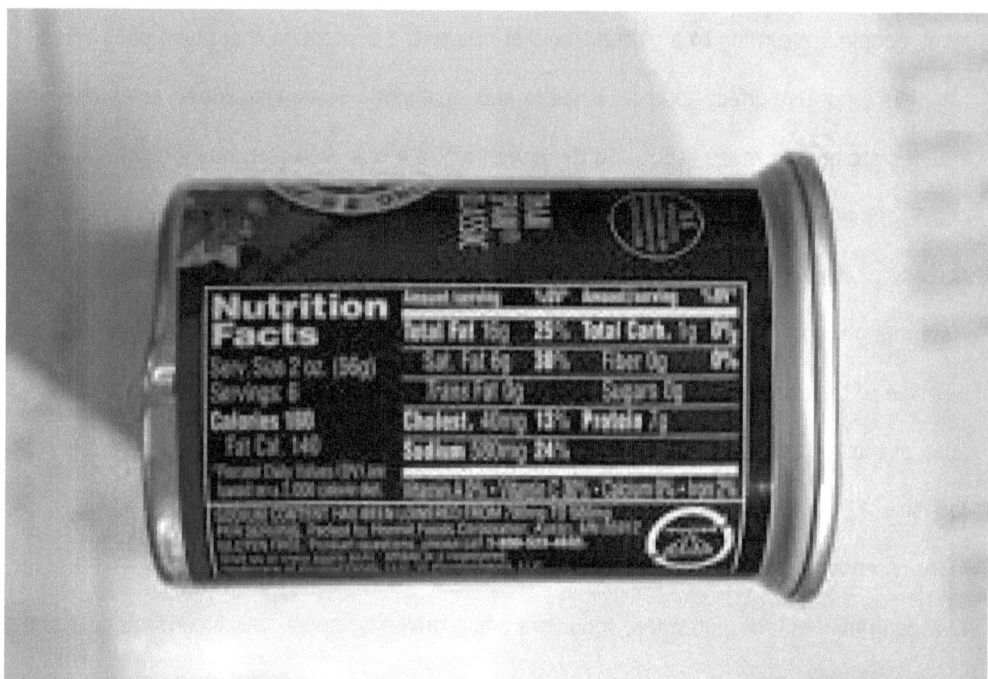

A recent survey by DuPont (Hamann, 2017) found that the most appealing food claims for consumers purchasing gluten free foods (apart from the gluten free claim) included claims that gluten free products contained high fibre, no added preservative, low saturated fat, low carbohydrates/calories and low sugar content.

Scientific evidence:

Many gluten free products are higher in fat and sugar and lower in protein and fibre than their gluten containing counterparts. There is no robust evidence that gluten free foods are more nutritious.

Study in 2015 of over 3,200 foods in Australia: A comprehensive study of over 3,200 gluten free and gluten containing foods was undertaken, examining the nutritional content of ten food groups including the core food groups of bread, pasta and breakfast cereals (Wu et al, 2015). The study compared the nutritional values of these gluten free products to their gluten containing counterparts.

The researchers found no significant differences in the nutritional values of the core food groups. Gluten free bread, pasta and breakfast cereals were not found to be more nutritious. Furthermore, their study revealed that these gluten free products had lower average protein content. Gluten free products in the discretionary food categories (which included cakes, biscuits, ice-cream, sausages, etc) were found to have slightly higher average nutritional values, but contained high levels of saturated fat, sugar and salt. The researchers concluded that overall, the consumption of gluten free products is unlikely to be more beneficial to the health of people who do not present with coeliac disease or gluten intolerance.

Summary

Over 3,200 products from 10 core food groups surveyed

- GF bread, pasta and breakfast cereals **not more nutritious**
- GF bread, pasta and breakfast cereals **lower in protein**
- GF cakes, biscuits, ice-cream, etc **high in saturated fat, sugar and salt**

Conclusion: **GF products unlikely to have health benefits** for those without coeliac disease or gluten intolerance

Study in 2015 of 189 foods in Austria: Research was also conducted on Austrian foods (Missbach et al, 2015) analysing the nutritional composition of 63 gluten free products and 126 gluten-containing counterparts from a range of food categories including flour, bread, pasta, cereals, cakes, biscuits and snacks.

This study found that:

Across all food categories, there was no difference between gluten free and gluten containing products with regard to carbohydrate, energy, fat, fatty acids, sugar and fibre content.

Across more than half of all food categories, the protein content of gluten free products was significantly lower (more than 2 times lower).

Overall, it was concluded that there are no additional nutritional health benefits to gluten free foods for healthy consumers.

Summary

189 products surveyed, including flour, bread, pasta, cereals, cakes and biscuits

- GF foods across all categories **no different** to gluten containing counterparts **for carbohydrate, energy, fatty acids, sugar and fibre**
- GF foods in more than half of the categories **significantly lower in protein**

Conclusion: **GF products offer no additional nutritional benefits** for those without coeliac disease or gluten intolerance

Study in 2018 of over 1700 foods in the United Kingdom: Similarly, a more recent study (Fry et al, 2018) analysed and compared the nutritional content of over 1,700 food products across ten food categories in the UK. These food categories included bread, flour, pasta, breakfast cereals, biscuits and crackers. The study focused upon fat, saturated fat, sugar, salt and protein content, comparing gluten free products with their regular counterparts. Where available, fibre content was also noted. The study revealed that gluten free products were significantly lower in protein content in nine out of the ten food categories, supporting the findings of the previous studies. Furthermore, differences in nutritional content were noted between gluten free and regular foods:

- More gluten free bread and flour products contained higher fat and sugar than regular products, apart from gluten free crackers.
- Gluten free products tended to have higher salt content than regular products.
- The fibre content of gluten free products was generally lower than regular products.

The researchers concluded that the nutritional differences observed between gluten free and regular products make it unlikely that the consumption of gluten free food could offer a healthy alternative diet to those who do not require it due to a medical diagnosis.

Summary

Over 1,700 products from 10 core food groups surveyed

- GF bread and flour **higher in fat and sugar**
- GF products across 9 food groups **significantly lower in protein**
- GF products have **higher salt content**
- GF products **generally lower in fibre**

Conclusion: **GF products unlikely to offer a healthier alternative diet** for those who do not require it due to a medical diagnosis

Some gluten free food can be junk food

Many gluten free products such as confectionery, snacks, and fried potato crisps/chips are still junk food – high in calories and low in nutritional value. A gluten free label does not magically transform them into healthy foods.

That said, if products such as bread, cakes and biscuits are replaced with salad, nuts and fruit options, the consumption of essential nutrients would increase, contributing to a healthier diet. A healthier diet can be followed without going gluten free.

Conclusions

The consensus amongst researchers is that there are no discernible nutritional benefits to replacing regular foods with their gluten free counterpart in the pursuit of a healthier lifestyle. Some gluten free products are higher in fat and sugar than their gluten containing counterparts. Many gluten free products have significantly less protein and the fibre content (where listed) was generally lower in gluten free products. Evidence based research that a gluten free diet is a healthier option is lacking (Gaesser and Angadi, 2012).

Does a gluten free diet enhance athletic performance?

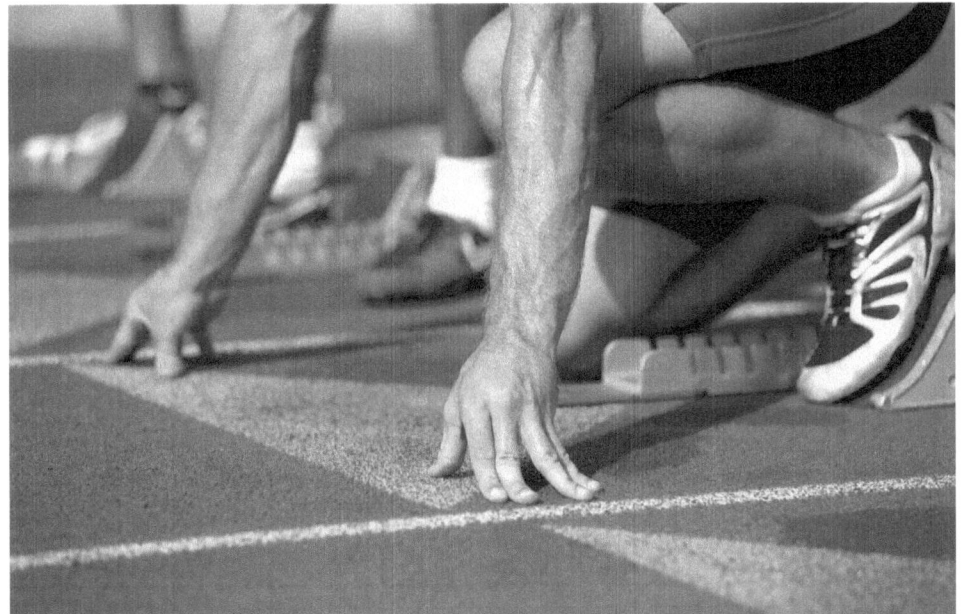

Popular belief:

A gluten free diet optimises athletic performance and prevents gastrointestinal

discomfort and distress.

Scientific evidence:

Studies so far have failed to demonstrate that a gluten free diet has positive effects

on athletic performance in those who do not have coeliac disease.

The gluten free diet has become very popular with athletes looking to improve their

performance and maintain good health. There are some athletes who follow the diet due to a diagnosis of coeliac disease. However, there are many more athletes who do not have a medical diagnosis, who are adopting the diet of their own volition.

How popular is the diet with athletes and why?

The extent of the popularity of the diet amongst athletes is illustrated in a 2015 international survey of over 900 non coeliac athletes (Lis et al, 2015), which revealed that:

- 41% of the athletes in the survey were following a GF diet more than 50% of the time (including some world and/or Olympic medallists).
- Of these, only 13% followed the diet for a reported medical condition.
- 57% of these athletes are self diagnosing gluten sensitivity and cite this as the primary reason for following a GF diet.

Only a small minority of athletes in the survey (13%) were following a gluten free diet due to a reported medical condition. Most adopted the diet with no medical based evidence for doing so.

The survey also revealed the main sources of information that the athletes relied upon for information about the gluten free diet.

Athletes' main sources of information and guidance on the gluten free diet (Lis et al, 2015)	
Online	28.7%
Trainer/coach	26.2%
Other athletes	17.4%

Those athletes who were regularly following a gluten free diet (more than 50% of the time) reported problems such as gastrointestinal symptoms and fatigue that were perceived to be caused by ingesting gluten, with 84% of these athletes reporting that their symptoms improved with the avoidance of gluten in their diet.

Celebrity athlete endorsements, alongside the perceived health benefits of a gluten free diet, contribute to its widespread adoption in the athletic world, with benefits linked to:

+ Enhancement of competitive performance
+ Reduction in gastrointestinal symptoms and inflammation
+ Overall better dietary health
+ A sense of wellbeing

But what is the scientific evidence?

Study in 2015: Randomised, double blind, crossover study of 13 non coeliac athletes

A study was undertaken to assess the effects of a gluten free diet on 13 non coeliac competitive endurance cyclists (Lis et al, 2015).

They were given a gluten free diet, alongside either gluten containing food bars or gluten free food bars for 7 days. After a 10 day washout period, they then crossed over. Their performance was assessed and blood samples were taken to analyze gastrointestinal symptoms.

The results did not show any significant differences between the gluten free diet and the gluten containing diet. The researchers concluded that a short-term gluten free diet had no overall positive benefits for non coeliac athletes.

Summary

Study of athletes and gluten free diet in 2015

- No significant difference in time trial performance whether on gluten containing or gluten free diet
- Gastrointestinal symptoms were similar on both diets
- No significant differences were observed with regard to inflammatory markers
- Wellbeing responses were similar on both diets

Conclusion: A short-term gluten free diet has no effect on performance, gastrointestinal symptoms, overall wellbeing or inflammatory markers

Clearly, athletes are experiencing perceived benefits from gluten exclusion, but with anecdotal evidence and self diagnosis, it is difficult to assess whether the effects can be solely attributed to gluten avoidance. So many other variables are involved, including making healthy food choices and also a belief that the diet is having a good impact – the placebo effect. The medical and scientific evidence to support these claims is scarce (Lis et al, 2015). Research would appear to indicate that, in fact, a gluten free diet does not enhance athletic performance.

Conclusions

There is a paucity of scientific research investigating the effects of gluten free diet upon athletic performance, so it is difficult to ascertain whether the diet does, in fact, has a positive impact upon performance. To date, the only study to assess the impact of a gluten free diet on athletes concluded that there were no beneficial effects of going gluten free on either performance or general health and wellbeing.

Does gluten cause heart disease?

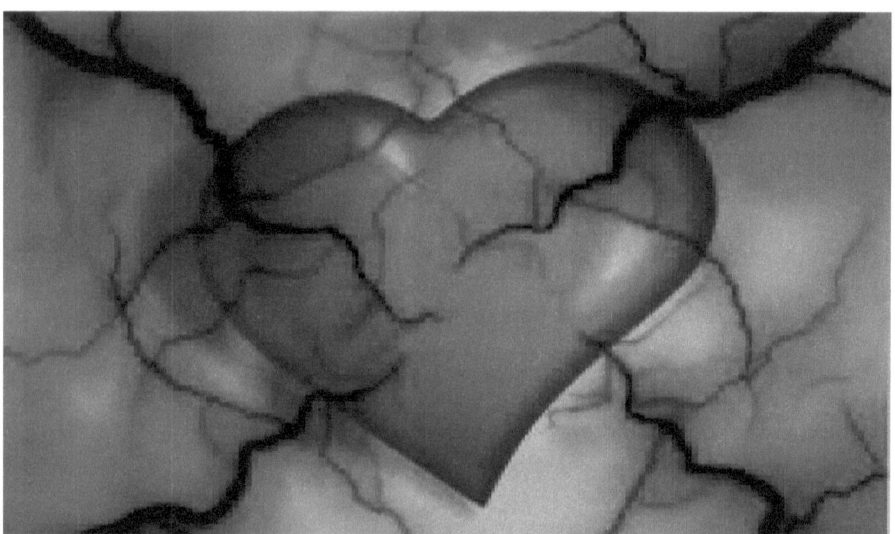

Popular belief:

Wheat is bad for you as it increases the risk of heart disease.

Scientific evidence:

A large number of scientific studies and trials have demonstrated that consuming wheat/gluten **does not** increase the risk of heart disease.

Wheat is alleged to be bad for you as it is claimed that it produces bad cholesterol and therefore increases the risk of heart (cardiovascular) disease. Eliminating wheat and grains from the diet eliminates bad cholesterol, according to anecdotal reports.

What are the risk factors for cardiovascular disease?

Cardiovascular diseases are the leading cause of death worldwide (British Heart Foundation, 2018).

The most significant risk factor for cardiovascular disease appears to be a higher number of small low density **lipoproteins** (LDLs) in the blood (Ivanova et al, 2017, Li et al, 2018). Lipoproteins are carrier proteins. They transport **cholesterol** around our body in our blood. Cholesterol is essential to our health and is both produced by our cells as well as produced through the foods we eat.

There are two types of lipoprotein:

High density lipoprotein (HDL) – absorbs cholesterol and takes it away to the liver to be flushed from the body. It is often referred to as 'good cholesterol'.

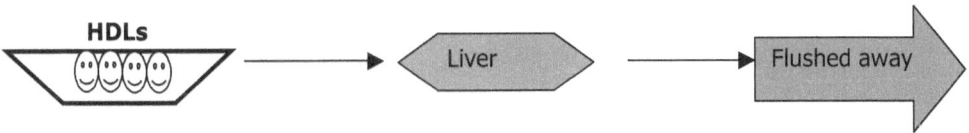

Low density lipoprotein (LDL): LDLs can be small, dense LDLs or large LDLs. Large LDLs are relatively desirable. Small LDLs, on the other hand, if in too great a quantity, can build up in the body and form plaque in the arteries, narrowing the vessels and restricting the blood supply to and from the heart. When the blood is blocked, it can cause angina or heart attack. Thus, LDL is often referred to as 'bad cholesterol'.

Small LDLs

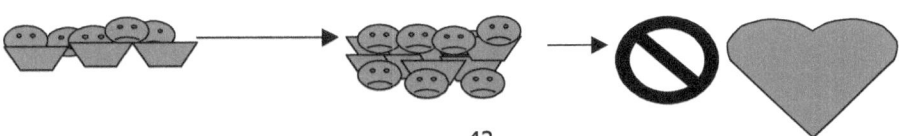

When cholesterol levels are assessed, three scores are normally given: HDL score, LDL score and overall combined score.

A higher level of HDL is seen as positive.

A higher level of LDL is seen as negative.

Diets high in carbohydrate are known to cause an increase in these small LDL particles – the bad cholesterol. As grains such as wheat contain carbohydrates, can it be concluded that wheat consumption causes heart disease?

Grains such as wheat contain carbohydrates. A high carbohydrate diet is known to cause an increase in bad cholesterol - small LDL particles. Should grains such as wheat be eliminated from our diet to avoid heart disease?

Scientific evidence

Wheat carbohydrates are no different to other carbohydrates.

Other carbohydrate types consumed in large amounts will also cause an increase in small LDL particles and therefore increase the risk of heart problems (Jones, 2012). The disappearance of small LDLs in patients who cut grains from their diet could be attributed to the reduction in overall carbohydrate consumption, rather than specifically from the avoidance of grains.

Study in 2012: Systematic review of 45 studies and 21 trials

A longitudinal study of 45 prospective cohort studies and 21 randomised controlled trials related to whole grain consumption and health outcomes between 1966 and 2012 was undertaken. Researchers found that those who consumed 3-5 servings per day (48-80g) of whole grains had a 21% lower risk of cardiovascular disease than those who rarely or never consumed whole grains (Ye et al, 2012).

> **Review of 45 studies and 21 trials found that eating 3-5 servings of whole grains per day reduced the risk of heart disease by 21%.**

Study in 2013: Systematic review and meta- analysis of 22 studies

22 cohort studies looking at the intake of dietary fibre and its association with heart disease were reviewed and analysed. The results indicated that diets containing high fibre, from cereal (grain) or vegetable sources specifically, were linked with a significantly lower risk of cardiovascular disease and coronary heart disease (Threapleton et al, 2013).

> **Systematic review of 22 studies found that diets high in fibre from cereal grains and vegetable sources significantly reduced the risk of heart disease.**

Study in 2016: 45 prospective studies

A meta-analysis of 45 studies was undertaken, analysing the effect that consuming particular amounts of whole grains had on a range of health issues including coronary heart disease and cardiovascular disease (Aune et al, 2016). The researchers found a 21% reduced risk of developing coronary heart disease and a 16% reduced risk of developing cardiovascular disease in those who consumed higher quantities of whole grains compared with those consuming low quantities of whole grains. It was concluded that a high intake of whole grains is linked with a reduced risk of cardiovascular disease.

> **Analysis of 45 studies concluded that the risk of developing coronary heart disease was reduced by 21% in those consuming higher amounts of whole**

Study in 2017 of over 100,000 participants over 25 years

A long term prospective cohort study of male and female health professionals without a history of coronary heart disease was undertaken, to assess whether long term intake of gluten was linked with the development of coronary heart disease. Over 100,000 participants' diets were monitored for over 25 years, looking at the quantity of gluten consumed and the incidence of coronary heart disease within the cohort. The researchers concluded that: '*Long term dietary intake of gluten was not associated with risk of coronary heart disease.*' (Lebwohl et al, 2017).

A 25 year study of over 100,000 participants found that:

Long term consumption of gluten **did not increase the risk** of coronary heart disease

Long term consumption of gluten **did not increase the risk** of having a heart attack

---

Conclusions

Any carbohydrates consumed in large amounts may increase the risk of developing heart disease. Wheat is no different to other carbohydrates in this respect. There is substantial scientific evidence that the consumption of whole grains does not increase the risk of heart disease. The weight of evidence indicates a reduced risk in those consuming higher amounts of whole grains. Long term consumption of gluten has not been found to increase the risk of heart disease. There is no credible scientific evidence to suggest that gluten should be avoided to reduce the risk of heart disease.

Does eating gluten cause diabetes?

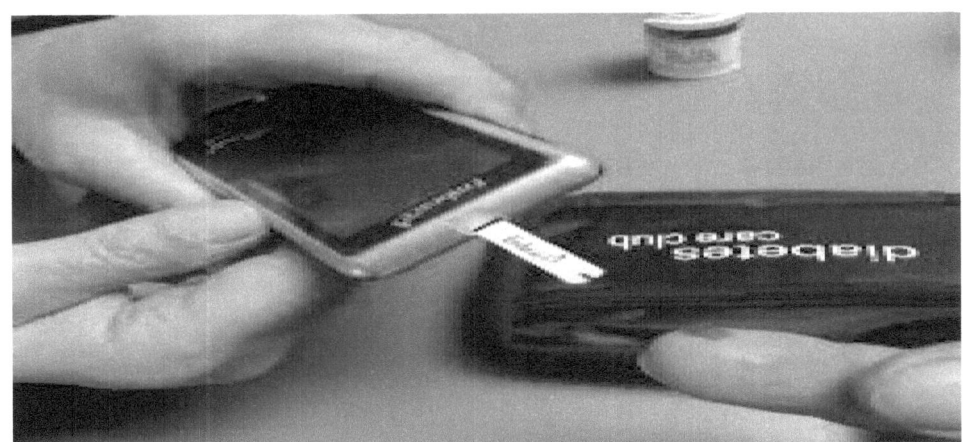

Popular belief:

Wheat is bad for you as it has a high glycaemic index (GI) and causes diabetes.

Scientific evidence:

The effect of food on our blood sugar levels is a complex interactive process between many different food components. The whole meal needs to be taken into account. Furthermore, studies have consistently found that moderate consumption of whole grains actually decreases the risk of diabetes.

Wheat, containing carbohydrate and having a higher glycaemic index (GI) than table sugar, is alleged to raise blood sugar to extremely high levels. High blood glucose damages cells in the pancreas responsible for the production of insulin. Repeated high blood glucose leads to insulin resistance and thus to diabetes. It is claimed anecdotally that diabetes has been cured in patients who have eliminated wheat from their diet (Davis, 2011).

What are the risk factors for diabetes?

Diabetes is a condition where people have too much glucose (sugar) in their blood. This leads to lots of different complications.

Everyone needs glucose for energy. Glucose is produced from the breakdown of carbohydrates that we ingest, which is then released into the bloodstream. Insulin is then needed to allow the glucose to pass from the bloodstream to our cells, providing us with the energy we need.

Insulin is produced by the pancreas. When glucose enters the bloodstream, the pancreas senses this and releases the correct amount of insulin to allow the glucose to transfer to our cells.

Type 1 diabetes means that a person cannot make any insulin.

Type 2 diabetes means that the insulin made isn't working effectively or there is not enough of it.

It is understood that there are several risk factors for diabetes, with no one singular cause. Risk factors include:

Genetics: Type 2 diabetes tends to run in families.

Obesity: Being overweight or obese sometimes causes insulin resistance, a precursor to type 2 diabetes.

Ethnicity: Type 2 diabetes occurs more often in particular ethnic groups.

Lack of exercise: Physical activity reduces blood sugar levels.

Diet: A healthy, balanced diet reduces the risk of developing type 2 diabetes.

Organisations such as Diabetes UK, The American Diabetes Association and the NHS are in general agreement on the risk factors for diabetes.

So what is the evidence that grains, specifically wheat - causes diabetes due to its high GI, and that the elimination of wheat in the diet eliminates diabetes?

Scientific evidence

Study in 2012: Review of 135 studies

An analysis of a total of 135 studies published between 2000 and 2010 were analysed, relating to the consumption of refined grains and health outcomes. Taking the totality of the evidence from all of these studies, it was concluded that the consumption of refined grains was not associated with increased risk of diabetes (Williams, 2012).

> **Review of 135 studies found no evidence to indicate that consuming refined grains increased the risk of diabetes.**

Study in 2012: Systematic analysis of 45 studies and 21 trials

A longitudinal study of 45 prospective cohort studies and 21 randomised controlled trials related to whole grain consumption and health outcomes between 1966 and 2012 was undertaken. Researchers found that those who consumed 3-5 servings per day (48-80g) of whole grains had a 26% lower risk of type 2 diabetes than those who rarely or never consumed whole grains (Ye et al, 2012).

> **Evidence from 45 studies and 21 trials found that the consumption of 3-5 servings of whole grains per day reduced the risk of type 2 diabetes by 26%.**

Study in 2013: Systematic review and meta-analysis of 16 studies

Sixteen studies were analysed to assess the link between whole grain consumption and type 2 diabetes. The researchers concluded: *'Our meta-analysis suggests that a high whole grain intake, but not refined grains, is associated with reduced type 2 diabetes risk.'* (Aune et al, 2013)

> **Review of 16 studies found that whole grain consumption was linked with a reduced risk of developing type 2 diabetes.**

Study in 2016: 45 prospective studies

A meta-analysis of 45 studies was undertaken, analysing the effect that consuming particular amounts of whole grains had on a range of health issues including diabetes. The researchers found *'a reduced risk of incidence of type 2 diabetes associated with up to two to three servings a day (60-90 g/day) of whole grain'*. They also found a reduction of 36% in the relative risk of death from diabetes in those who had a high rather than a low intake of whole grains. The researchers concluded that a high intake of whole grains is linked with a reduced risk of diabetes (and cardiovascular disease) (Aune et al, 2016).

> **Analysis of 45 studies found that consuming 2-3 servings a day of whole grains reduced the risk of developing type 2 diabetes.**

Can the GI index be misleading?

Taking account of GI is important in diabetes as different carbohydrates are digested and absorbed into the bloodstream at different rates. The GI Index tells us how quickly any carbohydrate food or drink will increase blood sugar levels when eaten. As too much sugar in the blood is not good, low GI foods can help to manage diabetes (Diabetes UK, accessed 20/5/18). However, just relying on the GI Index of an item of food is considered too simplistic as there are many factors that influence the effect that food has on our blood glucose levels (Diabetes UK, nd).

- Firstly, the whole composition of the food needs to be considered. The reason why table sugar has a relatively low GI is because it comprises:

50% glucose. This is high GI

50% fructose. This is low GI

The result is a moderate GI (Jones, 2012).

Both fat and protein lower the GI of a food (Diabetes UK, nd), which is why a Snickers bar, for example, has a relatively low GI. It contains fat. Fat slows down the absorption of carbohydrate. Snickers also contain nuts. Nuts are naturally low in GI. Snickers contain chocolate. The phenolics and antioxidants lower the GI of the candy bar. The result is that a Snickers bar has a calculated GI of 41 (Jones, 2012).

A quick glance at the GI Index of foods (Atkinson, et al, 2008) shows that:

Watermelon has a GI of 76

Spaghetti has a GI of 49

If we were to look at the GI Index of the foods alone, we could conclude from this that we should avoid watermelon and eat spaghetti instead!

However, if we eat the same portions of both of these foods, spaghetti will have a bigger effect on our blood sugar levels as it contains more carbohydrate than watermelon.

- Secondly, the effect of carbohydrate rich foods on blood sugar is affected by the amount of fibre in the food. Fibre slows down the process of carbohydrate absorption, therefore slowing the effect on blood sugar. High fibre foods include whole grains (Diabetes UK, nd).

- Thirdly, how the food is processed and prepared affects a food's GI. Typically, the more a food is subjected to heat and cooking, the higher the GI.

- Fourthly, it is important to consider what else is in the meal. It is advised that, rather than considering the GI value of a single item of food, the total GI index of a meal should be assessed, as other components of a meal may reduce the overall GI index.

In summary, the effect that food has on our blood sugar levels is a complex interactive process between many different food components (Diabetes UK, nd). The GI index alone can be very misleading.

The elimination of wheat from a diet may reduce an individual's overall carbohydrate consumption, which could lead to weight loss and thus result in the elimination of diabetes.

It is not disputed that weight loss is a recommended treatment for diabetes. However, a reduction in overall carbohydrate consumption, whether wheat based or not, would have a similar effect of reducing weight.

Conclusions

The weight of scientific evidence indicates that whole grain consumption is associated with a lower risk of developing type 2 diabetes. Reducing overall carbohydrate intake may reduce the risk, without eliminating wheat in particular. There is no research evidence that consuming wheat causes diabetes.

Marie Pendle-Clarke

Chapter 4

Is gluten free the key to a slimmer me?

Consumer surveys indicate that many people who adopt a gluten free diet are doing so in order to lose weight (Mintel, 2014, Hartman Group, 2015). The idea that a gluten free diet can help with losing weight has been fuelled by media reports of celebrities who have chosen to follow this diet, not for medical reasons, but in an effort to shed the pounds. Celebrities such as Lady Gaga, Miley Cyrus and Victoria Beckham have all reportedly adopted a gluten free diet.

Popular beliefs:

- A gluten free diet is healthier, lower in calories and can help to lose weight
- Wheat is a cause of obesity, so eliminating wheat eliminates obesity

Scientific evidence:

Gluten free products are not lower in calories than their gluten containing counterparts. Studies on those who have eliminated wheat/gluten from the diet have found that people are more likely to gain weight than lose weight.

Is a gluten free diet healthier and lower in calories?

The gluten free food industry has seen rapid growth in recent years, with the development of gluten free alternatives to anything from bagels and brownies to muffins and ice-cream. People perceive that these gluten free products can help with weight loss.

Scientific evidence

A study in Australia (2015) analysed over 3,200 gluten free and gluten containing foods of ten food groups including the core food groups of bread, pasta and breakfast cereals (Wu et al, 2015).

The researchers found no significant differences in the energy (calorie - kj) values of the core food groups. Gluten free bread, pasta and breakfast cereals were not found to be lower in calories.

Similarly, gluten free products in the discretionary food categories (which included cakes, biscuits, ice-cream, sausages, etc) were not significantly lower in calories, containing high levels of saturated fat, sugar and salt. The researchers warned that a gluten free label on a product can be misconstrued as healthier product. Summary:

Over 3,200 products from 10 core food groups surveyed
- GF bread, pasta and breakfast cereals **not lower in calories (energy/kj)**
- GF cakes, biscuits, ice-cream, etc **high in saturated fat, sugar and salt**

Research on Austrian foods analysing the nutritional composition of 63 gluten free products and 126 gluten-containing counterparts found that:

Across all food categories, there was no difference between gluten free and gluten containing products with regard to energy (Missbach et al 2015).

189 products surveyed, including flour, bread, pasta, cereals, cakes and biscuits

- GF foods across all categories **no different** to gluten containing counterparts **for energy (calories = kj)**

A recent study in the UK by Fry et al (2018) analysed and compared the nutritional content of over 1,700 food products across ten food categories in the UK. These food categories included bread, flour, pasta, breakfast cereals, biscuits and crackers. The study focused upon fat, saturated fat, sugar, salt and protein content, comparing gluten free products with their regular counterparts. Where available, fibre content was also noted. The study revealed that gluten free products were significantly lower in protein content in nine out of the ten food categories, supporting the findings of the previous studies. Furthermore, differences in nutritional content were noted between gluten free and regular foods:

- More gluten free bread and flour products contained higher fat and sugar than regular products, apart from gluten free crackers.
- Gluten free products tended to have higher salt content than regular products.
- The fibre content of gluten free products was generally lower than regular products.

The researchers concluded that the nutritional differences observed between gluten free and regular products make it unlikely that the consumption of gluten free food could offer a healthy alternative diet to those who do not require it due to a medical diagnosis.

Over 1,700 products from 10 core food groups surveyed

- GF bread and flour were **higher in fat and sugar**

The muffin bluff

An examination of a prominent UK supermarket's own brand of chocolate chip muffins, available in gluten containing and gluten free varieties reveals the following:

Ingredients of muffins	Gluten free muffin higher or lower than regular muffin?	Gluten free muffin contains...
Calories	⬆	Almost 10% more calories
Fat	⬆	Almost 20% more fat
Salt	⬆	Almost 35% more salt
Fibre	⬇	25% less fibre
Protein	⬇	Nearly 30% less protein

Source: www.sainsburys.co.uk

Conclusions

Scientific analysis of the content of gluten free foods in comparison to their gluten containing counterparts has demonstrated that they are generally higher in saturated fats, sugar and salt. The consensus amongst researchers is that there are no discernible benefits to replacing regular foods with their gluten free counterpart in order to be healthier. In fact, some gluten free products are higher in fat and sugar than their gluten containing counterparts.

The findings from these studies do not support the idea that a gluten free diet can help with weight loss.

Do we lose weight if we eliminate gluten and wheat?

There is a popular conception that wheat is a cause of obesity and therefore cutting out wheat results in weight loss.

An American study at the University of Iowa was cited (Davis, 2011) to support the claim

that eliminating wheat from a person's diet leads to weight loss.

The research was conducted at the Mayo clinic on 218 patients who had been diagnosed

with coeliac disease, looking at the effects of a gluten free diet on their symptoms. Analysis

of the effect of the diet on weight gave the following results (Murray, 2004):

After 6 months on a gluten free diet:

- **25 patients lost weight** (12 of whom had normal or low weight)

- **91 patients gained weight** within 6 months

- The percentage of **overweight males stayed the same**

- The percentage of **overweight females increased (from 14% - 17%)**

- The percentage of **obese males and females decreased**

Whilst the weight loss was most evident in those who were identified as obese at diagnosis,

it cannot be concluded from this data that avoidance of gluten results in weight loss.

A study in Northern Ireland (2006) (Dickey and Kearney, 2006) looked at 371 patients

with coeliac disease diagnosed over a 10 year period. Of these 371 patients, only 4% were

underweight at diagnosis.

188 of these patients who maintained a gluten free diet were assessed for weight gain after

two years of gluten exclusion. The researchers found that:

gained weight	⬆	81%
lost weight	⬇	15%
no change in weight	➡	4%

In patients who were **overweight at diagnosis:**

82% gained weight

The percentage of patients in the overweight category rose from 26% to 51%

Another study in Italy (2010) looked at 149 children and adolescents diagnosed with coeliac disease, of whom 77% were classed as healthy weight or overweight at diagnosis (Valletta and Cipolli, 2010). After 12 months on a gluten free diet, their BMI was again assessed.

A significant increase in overall BMI score for the children was observed.

The percentage of children who were overweight doubled from 11% to 21%.

Overall BMI score of children after 12 months gluten free	⬆
Percentage of children who were overweight	⬆

The researchers concluded that a gluten free diet appears to increase the risk of gaining weight and becoming obese.

For those patients who are underweight and malnourished at diagnosis, a gluten free diet is expected to lead to weight gain as the patient recovers and begins the process of re absorption of nutrients again. However, as was noted in Chapter 1, the classical 'failure to thrive' symptom of coeliac disease is much less common nowadays, with diagnosis often made in adulthood and other factors such as osteoporosis, family history, anaemia, etc. becoming important markers for identification, resulting in diagnosis before malnutrition develops (Valletta and Cipolli, 2010). Thus, some patients nowadays are overweight at diagnosis.

These studies indicate that a gluten free diet can actually increase body weight in coeliac patients who are overweight. Whilst this may be partly attributed to improved absorption of nutrients, it has also been evidenced that processed gluten free products contain higher levels of fats, sugar and salt.

The effect of gluten free diet on those without a medical diagnosis has not been established to date (Gaesser and Angadi, 2012), although a study on mice has been conducted (Soares et al, 2013).

6 mice were fed a very high-fat and low carbohydrate diet to promote obesity.

One group's diet contained 4.5% gluten. The other group's diet contained no gluten.

After 8 weeks:

- The mice on the **gluten free diet gained less body weight**
- The mice on the **gluten free diet showed reduced obesity**

  Researchers concluded gluten avoidance is beneficial in reducing weight gain

---

However, as with animal studies generally, it is not known whether the results would be replicated in humans. The very high fat, low carbohydrate diet is not typical of a human diet. Furthermore, it is not known whether the effects were specific to gluten or whether other protein content would produce the same result (Brouns et al, 2013). Caution is therefore advised in the interpretation of these results (ibid).

Summary

- Many gluten free products are higher in calories than their gluten containing counterparts, which will not aid weight loss
- Coeliacs on a gluten free diet have been shown to gain weight
- Reducing calorie intake can be achieved without the elimination of gluten
- Finding credible scientific studies indicating that gluten causes obesity and that a gluten free diet can help with losing weight is difficult.

Conclusions

A gluten free diet does not automatically lead to a reduction in the consumption of calories and therefore weight loss. The growth in the popularity of gluten free foods indicates that many people who are adopting the diet are replacing gluten containing items with their gluten free equivalents. Research has shown that these products typically contain more calories than their gluten containing equivalents. To mimic their gluten containing equivalent in terms of mouthfeel, ingredients such as sugar and fat are a frequent addition to gluten free products, thereby increasing the calorie content (Welstead, 2015). There is a lack of scientific evidence that gluten avoidance leads to weight loss.

However, eating fresh fruit, vegetables and nuts instead of biscuits, cakes and pastries is likely to lead to a reduction in the number of calories consumed. Avoiding the consumption of too many refined carbohydrate, high calorie foods can lead to weight loss, regardless of whether gluten is avoided.

Chapter 5

Sense and sensitivity – is the jury out?

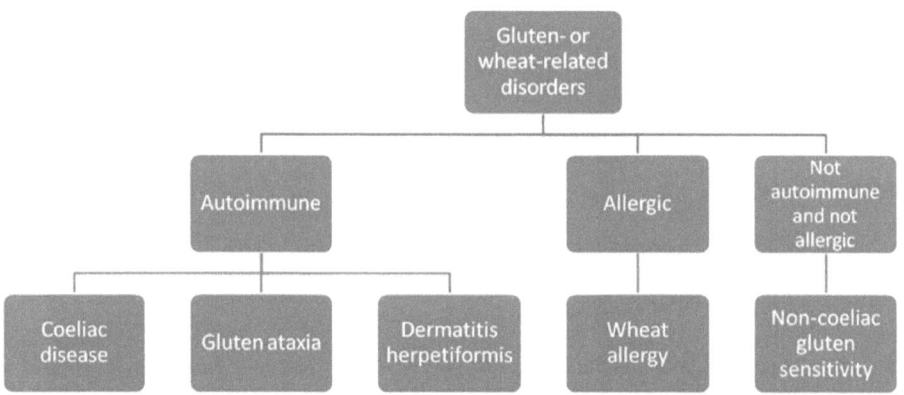

Biesiekierski (2017): The classification of gluten/wheat related disorders

Gluten sensitivity

The scientific community has recognised that there has been a significant increase in reported symptoms of sensitivity to gluten. As the vast majority of these patients do not have the traditional markers of coeliac disease, including damage to the intestinal mucosa induced by an autoimmune response to gluten, it was agreed to adopt the term 'non coeliac gluten sensitivity' in 2012.

With significantly increasing numbers of people presenting with apparent gluten sensitivity, questions have been raised about whether gluten is actually toxic for humans.

Are we just not able to tolerate gluten and grains?

Popular beliefs:

- Humans are not sufficiently adapted to the recent inclusion (in evolutionary terms) of wheat in our diets, making it toxic to our bodies.
- Recent wheat breeding practices are to blame for the rising incidence of gluten related disorders.

Scientific evidence:

- Archaeological evidence pinpointing when grains were introduced to the human diet is not conclusive.
- Studies have found no evidence that gluten/wheat is toxic in healthy individuals without coeliac disease.
- Research on wheat breeding practices is currently inconclusive. There is some evidence that we may be exposed to higher levels of gluten content in some modern wheat varieties, although there is also evidence of low gluten content in other varieties.

Eating like a caveman? The Paleo Diet

The hypothesis that humans are not adapted to grain consumption has led to the promotion of a stone-age or Palaeolithic (Paleo) diet as the key to good health.

The Paleo diet recommends removing all processed food from your diet - sugar, dairy and grains – the foods that our ancestors never consumed. It recommends eating non-processed meat, fish, eggs, fruit, vegetables, seeds and nuts. As the diet does not contain any grains, it is a naturally gluten free diet. It is argued that our genes are adapted to a pre-farming, pre-grain diet and that our stone-age ancestors did not suffer from heart disease, diabetes and autoimmune diseases on this diet (Cordain, 2011). Thus, avoiding grains and reverting to the diet of our ancestors can help to prevent many modern day illnesses and diseases.

The history of human grain consumption

It is commonly believed that the consumption of grass seeds began with the advent of agriculture, some 10,000 years ago. Prior to this Neolithic period, humans were understood to be hunter gatherers and believed to live on meat, nuts, roots and fruits (Aziz et al, 2015). Grains are therefore considered to be a relatively recent addition to the human diet, and the suggestion is that our bodies have not yet adapted to these changes.

However, whether the introduction of grains in the human diet occurred just 10,000 years ago is not firmly established. Evidence has emerged that humans may have been cooking and eating grains for far longer than has been generally assumed.

Researchers in Mozambique discovered grass seeds, including the sorghum grain, on tools dating back 105,000 years, during the Palaeolithic period (Mercader, 2009).

Researchers in 2010 reported finding grass seed starches in the teeth of Neanderthal skeletons from Iraq and Belgium (Henry, 2010). Furthermore, the seed starches showed markers indicative of having been cooked. This evidence suggests that the consumption of grasses was taking place over 100,000 years ago, during the Palaeolithic period.

A recent study (Arranz-Otaegui, 2018) found bread remains at a 14,000 year old hunter gather site in Jordan, with einkorn wheat, barley and oat cereal grains found. This discovery of the making and consumption of bread predates the emergence of Neolithic agriculture by 4,000 years.

The Stone Age

Palaeolithic	Mesolithic	Neolithic
Hunter gathering		Farming

Is gluten inherently toxic?

The idea that gluten is toxic to humans due to a lack of adaption to the consumption of grains is controversial and disputed by many in the scientific community.

An early study in 1966 (Levine) investigated whether the ingestion of large amounts of gluten (100-150g day) in healthy individuals over a period of time would have an effect upon absorption in the intestines or produce toxic effects upon the mucosa. The researchers found no evidence that a diet high in gluten had the toxic effect of producing lesions in the intestinal mucosa of healthy individuals.

> **Consumption of large amounts of gluten had no toxic effect on the intestines of healthy individuals.**

Similarly, a study in 1985 (Bramble) compared the effect that gluten ingestion had on a group of ten coeliac participants who had been on a gluten free diet for a minimum of 6 months and a group of four healthy participants with no history of coeliac disease (the control group). The results identified significant injury to the mucosa of coeliac patients, with the effects observed between 3.5 to 6 hours after being challenged with a singular high dose of gluten. In the control group, gluten toxicity was not induced with exposure to the same high level of gluten, with no injury to the mucosa evident. It was concluded that gluten sensitivity is exclusive to patients with coeliac disease.

> **Small scale study demonstrated that ingestion of gluten significantly injured the intestines of coeliac patients but was not toxic to non coeliac individuals.**

A more recent study in 2005 (Horiguchi) investigated the effects of wheat gluten on the immune systems of healthy individuals. A test group of 5 individuals was given 3g day of wheat gluten hydrolysate. A control group of 4 individuals was not given the wheat gluten. The results indicated no adverse effects to the wheat gluten.

> **No evidence that ingestion of wheat gluten had any adverse effect upon healthy individuals.**

Summary

The scientific evidence does not support the idea that gluten is inherently toxic and that it should be avoided. Studies have demonstrated that consuming large amounts of gluten did not produce adverse symptoms in healthy individuals.

Are we breeding Frankenwheat?

Wheat breeding practices have changed considerably over the years, responding to the need for efficient, large yield production of the grain. Breeding and selection has been systematically implemented to create higher yields and to produce varieties that are more disease resistant, adaptable to climate changes and have better bread making qualities. (Brouns, 2013). Does this mean that modern day wheat breeding is to blame for the apparent rise in gluten related disorders?

A study published in 2010 (Van den Broeck) investigated the differences between 36 modern European wheat varieties and 50 landrace (or ancient) varieties from all over the world. The researchers were looking for the presence of epitopes (the part of the molecule recognised by the immune system) known to cause an immunological response in people with coeliac disease. They found reduced genetic diversity of gluten proteins in the modern wheat varieties. A major epitope recognised by the majority of people with coeliac disease (Glia-_9) was more prevalent in modern wheat varieties than in the landrace varieties. The researchers concluded that modern wheat breeding may have increased the risk of exposure to epitopes linked to coeliac disease. However, it was also acknowledged that some modern varieties of wheat (and landraces) have been identified with quite low Glia-_9 epitope content.

A study published in 2013 (Kasarda, 2013) also investigated wheat breeding practices and the levels of gluten in modern day wheat varieties. After analysing available data, the researcher in this study concluded that there was no clear evidence of an increase in the gluten content of modern wheat varieties in the United States.

Conclusions

Archaeological evidence is not definitive about the date of introduction of grains into the human diet. It is possible that cereal grains have been part of the human diet for far longer than previously thought - long enough for us to have evolved and developed a tolerance for them.

However, even if it is accepted that grains are a relatively recent addition to the human diet in evolutionary terms, the argument that grains and gluten are toxic to humans has not been evidenced in scientific studies to date. Research into the effects of gluten consumption in healthy individuals has typically found no adverse effect upon the mucosal lining of the intestine that would indicate gluten's toxic effect on the body.

Studies analysing whether there is significantly increased gluten content in modern wheat varieties are currently inconclusive. More research is needed to form any convincing argument that modern wheat breeding practices have indeed created varieties of wheat with higher gluten levels likely to account for the apparent recent increase in gluten related disorders.

Non Coeliac Gluten Sensitivity

If, as the research evidence appears to suggest, gluten is not inherently toxic to healthy individuals, and we are more than likely sufficiently adapted to consuming grains in our diet, what does the scientific literature reveal about the condition non coeliac gluten sensitivity (NCGS)?

It is undeniable that many people experiencing gastrointestinal symptoms report feeling better on a gluten free diet, even though they do not have the established markers for coeliac disease (Mulder et al, 2013) or allergic symptoms. Symptoms such as abdominal pain, constipation, diarrhoea, fatigue and bloating are reported, mirroring the symptoms of coeliac disease. However, when tested, the genetic markers required for the development of coeliac disease (HLA – DQ2 or DQ8) are typically not present and neither is damage to the villi in the small intestine evident (Mulder, 2013, Aziz, 2015, Shewry and Hey, 2016).

This condition has been described as gluten sensitivity or gluten intolerance, but a recently accepted term of non coeliac gluten sensitivity has been introduced (Sapone et al, 2012). The condition is usually self reported by patients and confirmed following tests and the exclusion of other gluten related conditions (Aziz et al, 2015, Sapone et al, 2012). According to several surveys, perceived sensitivity or intolerance to gluten in the absence of coeliac disease is the most cited reason for adopting a gluten free diet. However, there is much controversy surrounding the idea that gluten can cause symptoms in people who do not have the characteristic intestinal damage of coeliac disease (Biesiekierski, 2017).

Is gluten to blame?

Studies have found that omitting gluten from the diet improved reported symptoms in people with NCGS. However, whether gluten is actually the culprit in producing coeliac disease like symptoms in people with NCGS has not been conclusively established within the scientific community (Aziz et al, 2015, Shewry and Hey, 2016).

A 4 week trial of 45 patients with irritable bowel syndrome (IBS) (where coeliac disease had been ruled out) at the Mayo Clinic were either on a on a gluten free diet or gluten containing diet. The results indicated that the omission of gluten in the diet led to an improvement in symptoms (Vazquez-Roque et al, 2013).

A study of 920 patients with symptoms of IBS and gluten sensitivity eliminated wheat from their diet and were challenged with wheat capsules. 30% of patients had no symptoms when excluding wheat and showed symptoms when ingesting wheat capsules. The researchers concluded that non coeliac wheat sensitivity is a distinct entity. However, it was acknowledged that it was difficult to conclude that gluten caused symptoms and that other components of wheat may be involved in inducing symptoms (Carroccio et al, 2012).

Although omitting gluten from the diet appears to alleviate symptoms, it is possible that other components of the grain could be implicated (Shewry and Hey, 2016). More specifically, research is indicating that it's possible that fermentable oligosaccharides, disaccharides, monosaccharides and polyols (FODMAPs) may be responsible for symptoms in people with NCGS, rather than the gluten protein of the grain (Biesiekierski, 2013).

A study in Australia (Biesiekierski et al, 2013) of 37 individuals with non NCGS was undertaken to assess the impact of gluten ingestion on their symptoms. It was hypothesised that if gluten was responsible for NCGS, then its ingestion would exacerbate symptoms and its avoidance would reduce symptoms. All participants followed a low FODMAP diet for two weeks initially, and then were given a high gluten, low gluten or gluten free diet. None of the participants knew which diet they were following, and each participant had a turn at each of the diets. The results of the study showed that:

- Introducing gluten to diets did not produce a specific response in most participants.
- Many reported a worsening of symptoms even when following a gluten free diet.
- All participants showed improved symptoms when on a diet low in FODMAPs.

Conclusion: **Gluten may not be a specific trigger for gastrointestinal symptoms in people with NCGS when the FODMAP content of diets is reduced.**

A recent study in Norway (Skodje, et al, 2017) investigated the effects of gluten and fructans on 59 non coeliac, non wheat allergy participants who were on a self imposed gluten free diet for self reported gluten sensitivity. Individuals were either given a placebo, gluten or fructans hidden in muesli bars, for seven days, in a double blind, placebo controlled crossover study. All participants completed all three challenges and were asked to report on their symptoms during each challenge. The results indicated that reported symptoms were at their highest when participants were consuming fructans, and significantly higher than when consuming gluten. It was concluded that fructans, rather than gluten, induced symptoms in individuals with self reported NCGS. Summary:

The overall symptom score was highest in individuals consuming fructans and significantly higher than those consuming gluten.

There was no difference in symptom scores between the gluten and placebo groups.

It was concluded that fructans, not gluten, induce symptoms of NCGS.

Are FODMAPS the answer?

FODMAPs such as fructans are a carbohydrate component in wheat and other grains. They are known to ferment very quickly and be poorly absorbed (Spiller, 2017), thus causing the gastrointestinal symptoms of gas and bloating. As bread and other wheat products contain FODMAPs, their consumption could prompt gastrointestinal symptoms. Likewise, omitting bread and wheat products from the diet could alleviate symptoms. It may not be the avoidance of gluten, but the avoidance of FODMAPs that improve symptoms.

The idea that FODMAPs rather than gluten could be implicated in NCGS has led to the suggestion that it should be renamed non coeliac wheat sensitivity (Carrochio et al, 2014).

However, FODMAPs are also found in other grains and in certain fruits and vegetables, so it may be misleading to refer only to wheat.

High FODMAP Foods (Monash University)

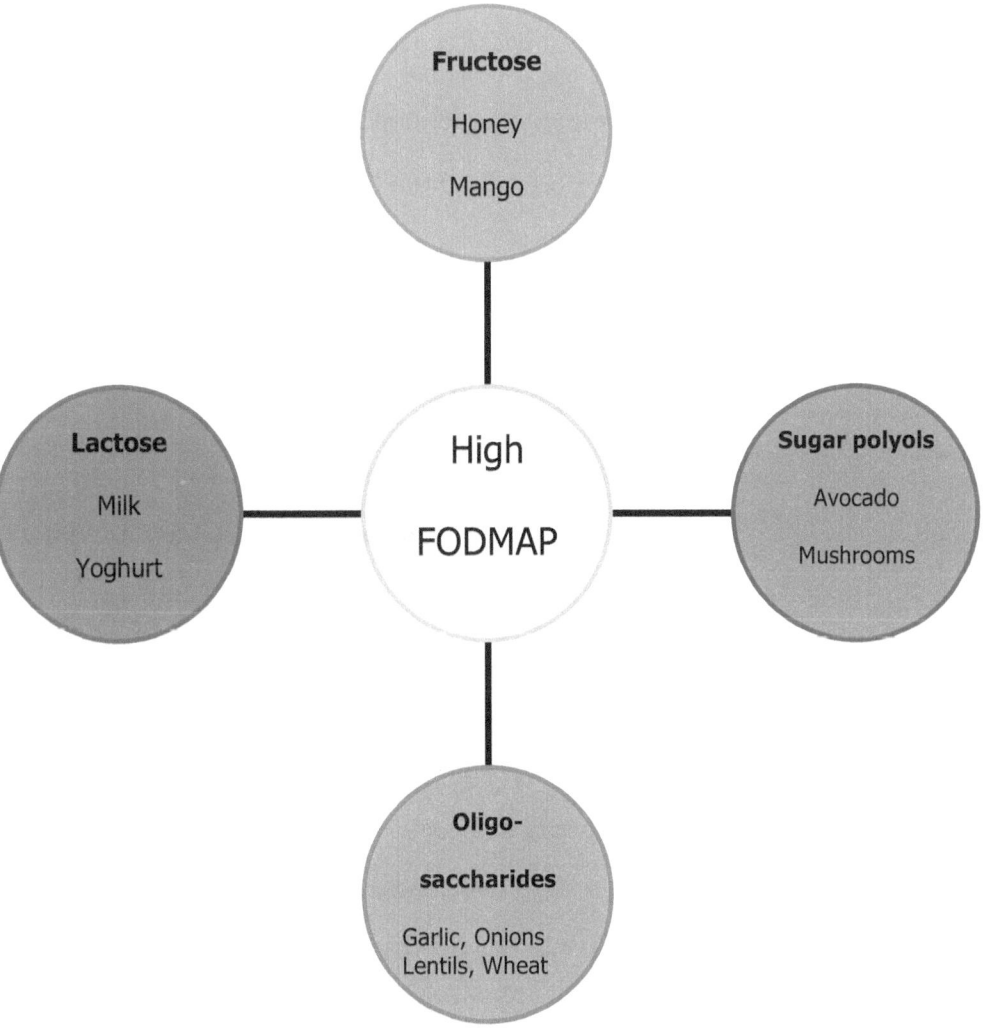

Research is still ongoing in this area, but the evidence to date is indicating that gluten may not necessarily be the factor causing the gastrointestinal problems in many people who report such symptoms, but rather that FODMAPs are implicated. This research appears to be little known, with the gluten free market substantially driven by consumers claiming gluten sensitivity.

Irritable Bowel Syndrome

Irritable bowel syndrome is characterised by gastrointestinal symptoms very similar to coeliac disease and non coeliac gluten sensitivity. A significant number of patients with CD are initially mistakenly diagnosed with IBS (El Salhy et al, 2015). It is therefore important that people presenting with IBS are screened routinely for coeliac disease (ibid).

There is an overlap between IBS and NCGS and it has been suggested that those with NCGS are a subgroup of patients with IBS (Catassi et al, 2013). Many patients with NCGS fulfil the diagnostic criteria for IBS. However, a study in 2012 found that non coeliac wheat sensitivity (NCWS) is a distinct clinical condition separate to IBS and that some patients who are diagnosed with IBS may actually have NCWS (Caroccio et al, 2012).

The effect of a gluten free diet on people with IBS is unclear (Catassi et al, 2013). Symptoms of IBS may be attributed to long-sugar-polymer-fructans rather than gluten (El Salhy et al, 2015) and a low FODMAP diet is considered to help alleviate the symptoms of IBS. (Aziz et al, 2015).

Conclusions

Unlike CD and IBS, there are, as yet, no diagnostic markers for NCGS. The debate also continues around the role of gluten in inducing symptoms of NCGS (Biesiekierski, 2017) and whether omitting gluten from the diet is the appropriate treatment. Given that most people

with NCGS are self diagnosed and put themselves on a gluten free diet with no medical

supervision (Catassi et al 2013), more research, clarity and communication about NCGS is

desperately needed. Going gluten free may not be the answer.

Marie Pendle-Clarke

Chapter 6

Is gluten free for you and me?

Should we complain about the grain?

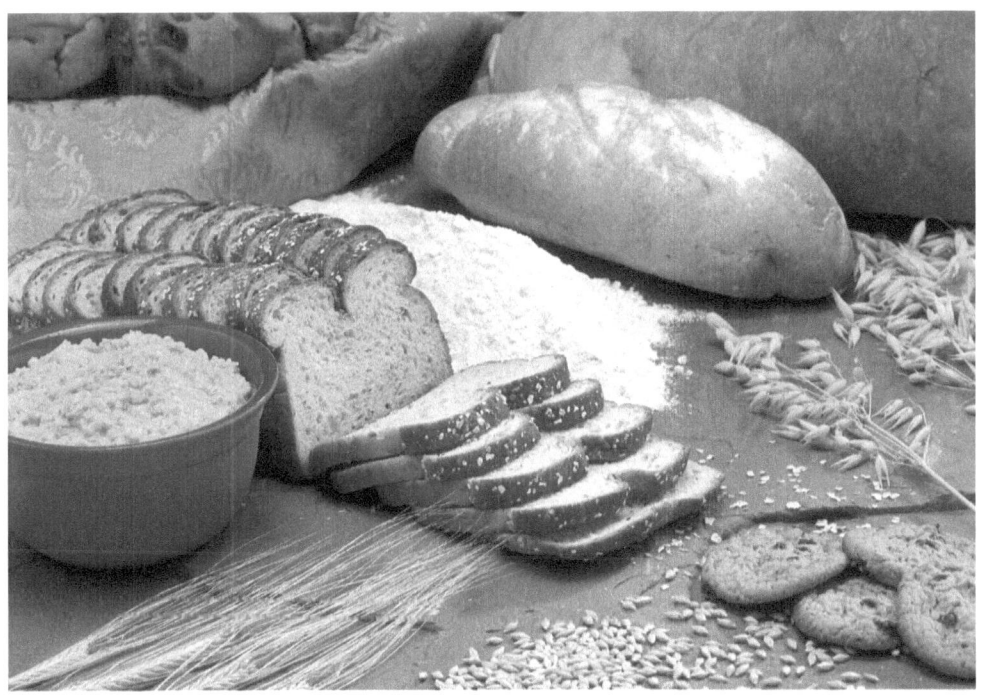

An examination of the current scientific evidence reveals no substantive evidence to suggest that a gluten free diet in people without coeliac disease is healthier, helps with weight loss or that we are not evolved to tolerate gluten.

What the science does reveal is that whole grain cereal products, which include those containing gluten, are rich in proteins, vitamins, minerals, carbohydrates, fats, oil and fibre. These compounds have very beneficial effects upon our health.

Are whole grains good or bad for our health?

A study in 2012 (Ye et al, 2012) analysed the results of 45 prospective cohort studies and 21 randomised controlled trials between 1966 and 2012. These studies compared the health outcomes of two groups:

1. Those who rarely or never consumed whole grains

2. Those who consumed 3-5 servings of whole grains a day (48-80g)

Overall, the results indicated that those people who consumed between 3 and 5 servings of whole grains per day has significantly lower risk of developing heart disease and diabetes. Furthermore, those who ate whole grains consistently gained less weight than those who rarely or never ate whole grains.

Summary:

---

45 prospective cohort studies and 21 randomised controlled trials over 46 years.

Compared with those who rarely or never consumed whole grains, those who consumed 3-5 servings of whole grains a day had:

- 21% lower risk of cardiovascular disease

- 26% lower risk of type 2 diabetes

- Consistently less weight gain over time (1.27kg v 1.64kg)

A study in 2016 analysed 45 prospective studies for the association between the amount of whole grains consumed and the risk of developing a range of diseases (Aune et al, 2016). Comparing the lowest levels of intake of whole grains with the highest intake levels, the results indicated that those consuming the highest levels of whole grains had a significantly reduced risk of developing coronary heart disease, cardiovascular disease or cancer and a

significantly reduced risk of death from respiratory disease, diabetes and infectious diseases.

Summary:

45 prospective studies

Compared with those with low levels of whole grain intake, those with high intake levels

had:

- 21% reduced risk of coronary heart disease

- 16% reduced risk of cardiovascular disease

- 11% reduced risk of total cancer

- 19% reduced risk of death from respiratory disease

- 36% reduced risk of death from diabetes

- 20% reduced risk of death from infectious disease

- 21% reduced risk of death from all non-cardiovascular, non-cancer causes

A study in 2017 involving long term observations of participants' diets through

questionnaires found that the risk of type 2 diabetes was increased in participants with low

levels of gluten intake (Zong, et al, 2017). The scientists concluded that limiting gluten in

the diet is less healthy due the lack of consumption of whole grains that are known to

reduce the risk of developing diabetes.

Properties of whole grains and effect on our health

Properties of whole grains	Found in	Effect on health	Lowers risk of
Antioxidants	Vitamins Phytochemicals Phenolic compounds	Protect against diseases	Cardiovascular disease Some cancers
Unsaturated fatty acid	Oleic and linoleic acid	Lowers blood cholesterol levels	Cardiovascular disease Type 2 Diabetes
Fibre	Fermentable carbohydrates Oligosaccharides	Reduces cholesterol Increases bowel transit time Increases gastric emptying rates Increases removal of carcinogenic compounds Helps with feeling fuller	Type 2 Diabetes Cardiovascular disease Obesity
Phytosterols	Sterols stanols	Inhibit absorption of cholesterol	Cardiovascular disease
Prebiotics	Oligosaccharides Resistant starches	Increase beneficial gut bacteria	Gastrointestinal inflammation Gastrointestinal cancers

Summary of scientific evidence

Systematic reviews and meta-analyses of a whole range of studies have consistently found that those who consume higher levels of whole grains in their diets have better health outcomes compared to those who do not consume whole grains.

- Lower risk of cardiovascular disease and coronary heart disease (Jonnalagadda et al, 2011, Ye et al, 2012, Threapleton, 2013, Aune et al, 2016)
- Lower risk of developing type 2 diabetes (Jonnalagadda et al, 2011, Ye et al, 2012, Aune et al, 2013, Aune et al, 2016)
- Lower body mass index (BMI), smaller waist circumference and less weight gain over time (Koh Banergee et al, 2003, Jonnalagadda et al, 2011, Ye et al, 2012)
- Improved digestive health (Jonnalagadda et al, 2011)
- Lower risk of developing certain cancers (Jonnalagadda et al, 2011, Aune et al, 2016)

For those with a diagnosis of coeliac disease, dermatitis herpetiformis or gluten ataxia, a gluten free diet is a must – it is the only way to stay healthy and prevent the body from having an adverse immune reaction to what is eaten. This group of people have a medically and scientifically evidenced adverse reaction to gluten.

For those with a wheat allergy, the avoidance of wheat is a must, to prevent an allergic reaction. This is also medically and scientifically evidenced.

For those with 'gluten sensitivity', the evidence is currently pointing strongly towards FODMAPS as the culprit rather than gluten. A gluten free diet may well minimise the symptoms, but this may be as a consequence of reducing FODMAPS rather than cutting out gluten. Following a low FODMAP diet may be a more effective, less restrictive and healthier solution, as other beneficial grains may still be included in the diet.

Self diagnosing and implementing a gluten free diet could actually be less healthy and do more harm than good, as people could be depriving themselves of essential fibre, vitamins and nutrients easily obtained from whole grains. Furthermore, adopting a gluten free diet without first undergoing medical investigations may, in some cases, disguise possible coeliac disease. Coeliac disease is much more difficult to detect once on a gluten free diet.

Whose interests are being served?

Despite popular social media, press and celebrity claims that gluten free is the way to be, credible evidence to support the claims just does not appear to exist. The rise in popularity of the diet appears to be driven more by consumer perceptions and commercial interests than by robust scientific evidence.

Many people rely upon processed foods for much of their diet and the cost of gluten free items is considerably more than their gluten containing counterparts (Fry et al, 2018). Sourcing and creating meals from alternative grains and flours that are gluten free, such as quinoa and teff, almond and coconut flour, are a challenge to people with busy lives and limited budgets.

There are issues surrounding compliance with the recognised threshold for the amount of gluten allowed in foods, issues with cross contamination and issues with general awareness and adherence to quality standards in restaurants to ensure the products served are gluten free.

It is not easy to follow a strict gluten free diet. A recent study (Syage et al, 2018) investigated the level of accidental gluten consumption in coeliac patients and found that adults with CD were on average accidentally consuming enough gluten to regularly induce symptoms and cause intestinal damage. Persistent ingestion of gluten in coeliacs can lead to other significant health complications. Good health therefore relies upon very strict adherence to gluten free standards, both inside and outside the home.

Improving health outcomes for the gluten free consumer

For consumers of gluten free products to maintain good health, there needs to be a concerted effort to improve the nutritional content of the foods. Lack of fibre in many products is a major concern given the importance of fibre in the prevention of chronic diseases such as cardiovascular disease and some cancers. Similarly, the higher levels of sugar and fat in the products need to be reviewed, to help address issues of obesity and diabetes. Lack of vitamin and mineral enrichment and fortification also leaves many consumers lacking in essential nutrients in their diet.

More research is needed into whether it is possible to produce a variety of oats that is completely free of the protein that causes a reaction in some coeliacs. Whilst most coeliacs can apparently tolerate gluten free, uncontaminated oats, there are a small minority that cannot, further reducing the opportunities for whole grain consumption.

Eating out should be worry free from a health and safety perspective. Consumers do not expect to become ill from e-coli or salmonella. Similarly, coeliacs should not expect to become ill from gluten contamination. If food outlets are offering gluten free options to attract customers, there are responsibilities attached to this, including strict compliance with gluten free standards and comprehensive staff awareness, from chef to serving staff.

If the food industry is happy to profit from the rise in the popularity of the gluten free diet, it is incumbent upon all involved to take seriously the health issues of those for whom a gluten free diet can be a matter of life or death, and also to prioritise the interests of their consumers looking for healthier alternatives.

Is anyone listening to the scientists?

Of the many factors influencing consumers of gluten free food, scientific research does not appear to figure very highly. But can we afford to ignore it? Below are just some of the conclusions reached by scientists through rigorous research.

- *'Current scientific evidence indicates that whole grains play an important part in lowering the risk of chronic diseases, such as coronary heart disease, diabetes and cancer, and also contribute to body weight management and gastrointestinal health.'* *(Jonnalagadda, 2011)*

- *'...evidence-based research supporting the merits of a gluten free diet as a healthier option for the general population is lacking.' (Gaesser et al, 2012)*

- *'...our systematic review and meta-analysis of 45 prospective cohorts and 21 randomized intervention trials indicates that increased intake of whole grain and fiber may lower the risk of T2D, CVD, and weight gain. Our findings support current recommendations stating that consumption of at least 48 g whole grains/d (approximately 3 servings/d) may offer beneficial effects for weight maintenance and the prevention of vascular disease' (Ye et al, 2012)*

- *'Since most of the evidence against wheat or gluten is unsubstantiated by science, there is no need for patients to avoid gluten unless they have celiac disease...'* (Cadenhead and Sweeny, 2013)

- *'There is strong evidence from prospective cohort studies that increased intakes of total dietary fibre, and particularly cereal fibre and wholegrain, as they are classified in this report, are associated with a lower risk of cardio-metabolic disease and colo-rectal cancer.'* (Scientific Advisory Commission on Nutrition 2015)

- *'For individuals who do not have CD, wheat allergy, or NCGS...there are no data supporting the presumed health benefits of a GFD. In fact, the opposite may be true in certain cases, particularly when the diet is followed without the guidance of an experienced registered dietitian or physician.'* (Reilly, 2016)

- *'This meta-analysis provides further evidence that whole grain intake is associated with a reduced risk of coronary heart disease, cardiovascular disease, and total cancer, and mortality from all causes, respiratory diseases, infectious diseases, diabetes, and all non-cardiovascular, non-cancer causes. These findings support dietary guidelines that recommend increased intake of whole grain to reduce the risk of chronic diseases and premature mortality.'* (Aune, et al, 2016)

****

Conclusions

Cardiovascular disease, diabetes, cancer and obesity are currently major threats to our health and longevity in this modern age, despite an apparently increasing consumer appetite for so called healthier foods and improved ways of living. Of concern are the sources of information upon which many people base their lifestyle decisions, which include the media (celebrities, sportspeople and bloggers), friends and family recommendations and health trends. Sportspeople have been reported to go online, take advice from their trainer/coach or listen to advice from other athletes when making dietary choices. It seems few people are taking notice of credible scientific research.

Scientists have demonstrated ways in which we can reduce our risk of developing these chronic diseases. Overwhelmingly, the weight of scientific evidence advises against avoiding gluten in the diet of healthy individuals. A diet rich in whole grains has been repeatedly shown to have positive health effects, reducing the risk of developing heart disease, cancer and diabetes, and contributing to good weight management when incorporated as part of a balanced diet.

The challenge now, it seems, is in communicating this research to the health conscious consumer, so that we can all make informed, scientifically evidenced, robust choices about how to improve and maintain our own health and wellbeing.

References

Adams, J. (2017) *Report Charts Global Gluten-free Market Growth Through 2023.* Celiac.com. Accessed 5/6/18 at https://www.celiac.com/articles.html/miscellaneous-information-on-celiac-disease/conferences-publicity-pregnancy-church-bread-machines-distillation-beer/report-charts-global-gluten-free-market-growth-through-2023-r4049/.

American Diabetes Association (nd) *Lower Your Risk.* Accessed 3/5/18 at http://www.diabetes.org/are-you-at-risk/lower-your-risk/?loc=atrisk-slabnav.

Arranz-Otaeguia, A.; Carreterob, L.G.; Ramsey, M.N.; Fuller, D.Q. and Richtera, T. (2018) Archaeobotanical evidence reveals the origins of bread 14,400 years ago in northeastern Jordan. *Proceedings of the National Academy of Sciences* Accessed 18/7/18 at www.pnas.org/cgi/doi/10.1073/pnas.1801071115.

Atkinson, F.S.; Foster-Powell, K. and Brand-Miller, J.C. (2008) International tables of glycemic index and glycemic load values: 2008. *Diabetes Care* 31, 12, 2281-2283. Available from http://care.diabetesjournals.org/content/diacare/31/12/2281.full.pdf

Aune, D., Keum N.; Giovannucci E.; Fadnes, L. *et al (2016)* Whole grain consumption and risk of cardiovascular disease, cancer, and all cause and cause specific mortality: systematic review and dose-response metaanalysis of prospective studies. *BMJ 53* i2716. doi:10.1136/bmj.i2716.

Aune, D.; Romundstad, P. and Vatten, L.J. (2013) Whole grain and refined grain consumption and the risk of type 2 diabetes: a systematic review and dose–response meta-analysis of cohort studies. *European Journal of Epidemiology 28*, 11, 845–858.

Aziz, I.; Branchi, F. and Sanders, D.S. (2015) The rise and fall of gluten! Conference on 'Carbohydrates in Health: friends or foes', Plenary Lecture 3: Waterlow lecture, *Proceedings of the Nutrition Society 74*, 221–226.

Aziz, I.; Karajeh, M.A.; Zilkha, J.; Tubman, E.; Fowles C. and Sanders, D.S. (2014) Change in awareness of gluten-related disorders among chefs and the general public in the UK: a 10-year follow-up study. *European Journal of Gastroenterology and Hepatology 26*, 11, 1228-33.

Benoit, L.; Masiri, J.; del Blanco, I.A.; Meshgi, M.; Gendel, S.M. and Samadpour, M. (2017) Assessment of Avenins from Different Oat Varieties Using R5-Based Sandwich ELISA. *Journal of Agricultural and Food Chemistry 65*, 8, 1467–1472.

Biesiekierski, J.R. (2017) What is Gluten? *Journal of Gastroenterology and Hepatology 32*, 1, 78–81.

Biesiekierski, J.R.; Peters, S.L.; Newnham, E.D.; Rosella, O.; Muir, J.G. and Gibson, P.R. (2013) No effects of gluten in patients with self-reported non-celiac gluten sensitivity after dietary reduction of fermentable, poorly absorbed, short-chain carbohydrates. *Gastroenterology 145*, 320–328.

Bramble, M. G.; Zucoloto, S.; Wright, N. A. and Record, C .O. (1985) Acute gluten challenge in treated adult coeliac disease: a morphometric and enzymatic study. *Gut 26*, 169-174.

British Heart Foundation (2018) *UK Factsheet* August 2018, PDF.

Brouns, F.J.P.H; van Buul, V.J. and Shewry, P.R. (2013) Does wheat make us fat and sick? *Journal of Cereal Science 58*, 209-215.

Bustamante, M.A.; Fernández-Gil, M.P.; Churruca, I.; Miranda, J.; *et al* (2017) Evolution of Gluten Content in Cereal-Based Gluten-Free Products: An Overview from 1998 to 2016, *Nutrients 9* ,1, 21.

Cadenhead, K. and Sweeny, M. (2013) Gluten elimination diets: Facts for patients on this food fad. *Council on Health Promotion Nutrition Committee, BC Medical Journal 55*, 3.

Carroccio A.; Mansueto P.; Iacono G.; Soresi, M.; et al. (2012) Non-celiac wheat sensitivity diagnosed by double-blind placebo-controlled challenge: exploring a new clinical entity. *American Journal of Gastroenterology 107*, 1898–1906.

Carroccio, A.; Rini, G. & Mansueto, P. (2014) Non-celiac wheat sensitivity is a more appropriate label than nonceliac gluten sensitivity. *Gastroenterology 146*, 320–321.

Catassi, C.; Bai, J.C.; Bonaz B.; Bouma, G.; *et al (2013)* Non-Celiac Gluten sensitivity: the new frontier of gluten related disorders. *Nutrients 26,* 5, 3839–53.

Celiac Disease Foundation (2014), *Oats and the gluten free diet.* Accessed 1/5/18 at

https://celiac.org/about-the-foundation/featured-news/2014/12/oats-and-gfd/.

Coeliac New Zealand *Gluten free and low gluten standards- NZ & Australia.* Accessed

3/7/18 at https://www.coeliac.org.nz/health-professionals-low-gluten.

Coeliac UK (2015) *Update on gluten-free product recall*, Accessed 23/9/18 at

https://www.coeliac.org.uk/about-us/news/update-on-gluten-free-product-recall/.

Coeliac UK (nd) *Dermatitis Herpetiformis*. Accessed 22/5/18 at

https://www.coeliac.org.uk/coeliac-disease/about-coeliac-disease-and-dermatitis-

herpetiformis/dermatitis-herpetiformis/.

Coeliac UK (nd) *Law on Gluten Free*. Accessed 3/7/18 at https://www.coeliac.org.uk/gluten-

free-diet-and-lifestyle/food-shopping/law-on-gluten-free/.

Coeliac UK (nd) *Neurological conditions*. Accessed 23/5/18 at

https://www.coeliac.org.uk/coeliac-disease/about-coeliac-disease-and-dermatitis-

herpetiformis/neurological-conditions/.

Coeliac UK (nd) *Oats*   Accessed 1/5/18 at https://www.coeliac.org.uk/gluten-free-diet-and-

lifestyle/gf-diet/oats/.

Coeliac UK (nd), *Catering and the law*. Accessed 8/6/18 at https://www.coeliac.org.uk/food-

industry-professionals/gluten-free-and-the-law/catering-and-the-law/.

Coeliac UK: (nd) *Myths about coeliac disease*. Accessed 3/7/18 at

https://www.coeliac.org.uk/coeliac-disease/myths-about-coeliac-disease/.

Collin, P.; Thorell, L.; Kaukinen, K. and Maki, M. (2004) The safe threshold for gluten contamination in gluten-free products. Can trace amounts be accepted in the treatment of coeliac disease? *Alimentary Pharmacology and Therapeutics 19*, 12, 1277-83.

Copping, A.M. (1978) The History of the Nutrition Society, *Proceedings of the Nutrition Society 37*, 105–139. Accessed 3/5/18 at

https://www.cambridge.org/core/journals/proceedings-of-the-nutrition-society/article/history-of-the-nutrition society/FEBE28C5D984EAE32C73D92E3CD0C608

Cordain, L. (2011) *The Paleo Diet: Lose Weight and Get Healthy by Eating the Foods You Were Designed to Eat*. New Jersey, Wiley and Sons.

Creed, T. (2016) *No, oats are not gluten free – here's why*. Blog. Accessed 1/5/18 at

https://www.ceres.co.nz/blog/no-oats-are-not-gluten-free-heres-why/.

Davis, W. (2011) *Wheat Belly: Lose the Wheat, Lose the Weight, and Find Your Path Back to Health*, New York, Rodale, Inc.

Diabetes UK (nd) *Diabetes Risk Factors*. Accessed 3/5/18 at

https://www.diabetes.org.uk/preventing-type-2-diabetes/diabetes-risk-factors .

Diabetes UK (nd) *Glycaemic Index and Diabetes*. Accessed 20/5/18 at

https://www.diabetes.org.uk/guide-to-diabetes/enjoy-food/carbohydrates-and-

diabetes/glycaemic-index-and-diabetes.

Dickey, W. and Kearney, N. (2006) Overweight in Celiac Disease: Prevalence, Clinical

Characteristics, and Effect of a Gluten-Free Diet. *American Journal of Gastroenterology 101*,

2356–2359.

El-Salhy, M.; Hatlebakk, J.G.; Gilja, O.H. and Hausken, T. (2015) The relation between celiac

disease, nonceliac gluten sensitivity and irritable bowel syndrome. *Nutrition Journal 14*, 92.

Fletcher, J. (2018) *What happens in gluten ataxia?* Accessed 22/5/18 at

https://www.medicalnewstoday.com/articles/320730.php.

Food and Drug Administration (2018) *Questions and Answers: Gluten-Free Food Labeling
Final Rule*. Accessed 1/8/18 at

https://www.fda.gov/Food/GuidanceRegulation/GuidanceDocumentsRegulatoryInformation/

Allergens/ucm362880.htm#Gluten_Levels.

Fric, P.; Gabrovska, D. and Nevoral, J. (2011) Celiac disease, gluten-free diet, and oats

*Nutrition Reviews 6*9, 2, 107-115.

Fry, L.; Madden, A. & Fallaize, R. (2018) An investigation into the nutritional composition

and cost of gluten free versus non-gluten free food products in the UK. *Journal of Human

Nutrition and Dietetics 31*, 1, 108-120.

Gaesser, G.A. and Angadi, S.S. (2012) Gluten-Free Diet: Imprudent Dietary Advice for the General Population? *Journal of the Academy Of Nutrition and Dietetics 112*, 9.

Gilissen, L.J.W.J.; van der Meer, I.M. and Smulders, M.J.M. (2016) Why Oats Are Safe and Healthy for Celiac Disease Patients. *Medical Sciences, 4,* 21.

Giménez, M.J.; Real, A.; García-Molina, M.D.; Sousa, C. and Barro, F. (2017) Characterization of celiac disease related oat proteins: bases for the development of high quality oat varieties suitable for celiac patients, *Scientific Reports* 7, 42588.

Grand View Research (2017*) Gluten-Free Products Market Analysis by Product (Bakery, Dairy Alternatives, Desserts & Ice-Creams, Prepared Foods, Pasta & Rice), By Distribution (Grocery Stores, Mass Merchandiser, Club Stores), and Segment Forecasts, 2018 – 2025*: Report Summary. Accessed 11/7/18 at https://www.grandviewresearch.com/industry-analysis/gluten-free-products-market.

Halmos, E.P.; Di Bella, C.A.; Webster, R.; Deng, M. and Tye-Din, J.A. (2018) Gluten in "gluten-free" food from food outlets in Melbourne: a cross-sectional study. *The Medical Journal of Australia 209*, 1.

Hamann, L. (2017) *Insights into the real gluten free needs and expectations of UK consumers.* DuPont Nutrition and Health BSB Autumn Conference, 11 October.

Hendrie, G., Baird, D., Golley, S. and Noakes, M. (2016) CSIRO Healthy Diet Score 2016, *Commonwealth Scientific and Industrial Research Organisation* (CSIRO).

Henry, A.G.; Brooks, A.S. and Piperno, D.R. (2011) Microfossils in calculus demonstrate consumption of plants and cooked foods in Neanderthal diets (Shanidar III, Iraq; Spy I and II, Belgium). *Proceedings of the National Academy of Sciences, 108*, 2, 486-491.

Horiguchi N., Horiguchi H. and Suzuki Y. (2005) Effect of wheat gluten hydrolysate on the immune system in healthy human subjects. *Bioscience, Biotechnology*, and *Biochemistry 69*, 2445-9.

Ivanova, E.A.; Myasoedova, V.A.; Melnichenko, A.A; Grechko, A.V. and Orekhov, A.N. (2017) Small dense low-density lipoprotein as biomarker for atherosclerotic diseases. *Oxid Med Cell Longev.* 1273042.

Janatuinen, E.K.; Kemppainen, T.A; Julkunen, R.J.K.; Kosma, V-M.; *et al* (2002) No harm from five year ingestion of oats in coeliac disease. *Gut 50,* 332–5.

Jones, J. (2012) Wheat Belly: An Analysis of selected Statements and Basic Theses from the Book, *Cereal Foods World 57*, 4, 177-189.

Jonnalagadda, S.S.; Harnack, L.; Liu, R.H.; McKeown, N.; *et al* (2011) Putting the Whole Grain Puzzle Together: Health Benefits Associated with Whole Grains—Summary of American Society for Nutrition 2010 Satellite Symposium. *The Journal of Nutrition 141*, 1011S–1022S.

Kasarda, D.D. (2013) Can an increase in celiac disease be attributed to an increase in the gluten content of wheat as a consequence of wheat breeding? *Journal of Agricultural and Food Chemistry 61*, 1155-9.

Koerner, T.B.; Cleroux, C.; Poirier, C.; Cantin, I.; *et al* (2013) *Gluten contamination of naturally gluten-free flours and starches used by Canadians with celiac disease.* Food Addit. Contam. Part A Chem. Anal. Control Expo. Risk Assess. *30*, 2017–2021.

Koh-Banerjee, P.; Franz. M.; Sampson, L.; Liu, S.; *et al* (2004) Changes in whole-grain, bran, and cereal fiber consumption in relation to 8-y weight gain among men. *The American Journal of Clinical Nutrition 80*, 5, 1237-45.

Lebwohl B.; Cao Y.; Zong G.; Hu, F.; *et al* (2017) Long term gluten consumption in adults without celiac disease and risk of coronary heart disease: prospective cohort study. *BMJ* 357:j1892.

Lee, H.J.; Anderson, Z. and Ryu, D. (2014) Gluten Contamination in Foods Labeled as "Gluten Free" in the United States, *Journal of Food Protection 77*, 10, 1830–1833.

Lerner, A.; Jeremias, P. and Matthias, T. (2015) The World Incidence Of Celiac Disease Is Increasing: A Review. *International Journal of Recent Scientific Research 6*, 7, 5491-5496.

Levine, R.A.; Briggs, G.W.; Harding, R.S. and Nolte, L.B. (1966) Prolonged gluten administration in normal subjects. *New England Journal of Medicine 274*, 1109-14.

Li, G., Wu, H. K., Wu, X. W., Cao, Z., *et al* (2018) Small dense low density lipoprotein-cholesterol and cholesterol ratios to predict arterial stiffness progression in normotensive subjects over a 5-year period. *Lipids in Health and Disease 17*, 1, 27. doi:10.1186/s12944-018-0671-2.

Lis, D. M., Stellingwerff, T., Shing, C. M., Ahuja, K. D. K., & Fell, J. W. (2015) Exploring the Popularity, Experiences, and Beliefs Surrounding Gluten-Free Diets in Nonceliac Athletes. *International Journal of Sport Nutrition and Exercise Metabolism 25*, 1, 37–45.

Lis, D., Stellingwerff, T., Kitic, C. M., Ahuja, K. D. K., & Fell, J. (2015) No Effects of a Short-Term Gluten-free Diet on Performance in Nonceliac Athletes. *Medicine & Science in Sports & Exercise 47,* 12, 2563-2570.

Lundin, K.E.A.; Nilsen, E.M.; Scott, H.G.; Løberg, E.M.; *et al* (2003) Oats induced villous atrophy in coeliac disease. *Gut 52*, 1649–1652.

Maglio M., Mazzarela G., Barone M. V., Gianfrani, C.; *et al* (2011) Immunogenecity of two oat varieties in relation to their safety for celiac patients. *Scandinavian Journal of Gastroenterology 46*, 1194–1205.

Mascaraque, M. (2018) *What the New Health and Wellness Data is Telling Us: A Look into Latest Trends.* Accessed 11/7/18 at https://blog.euromonitor.com/2018/02/new-health-wellness-data-look-latest-trends.html .

Mercader, J. (2009) Mozambican Grass Seed Consumption During the Middle Stone Age. *Science* 326, 5960, 1680-1683.

Miller, K. (2016) *How to Cater for Customers Following Gluten Free Diets*. Accessed 30/9/18 at https://www.bighospitality.co.uk/Article/2016/05/09/How-to-cater-for-customers-following-gluten-free-diets .

Mintel (2016) *Free-from gains momentum: Sales of free-from food products forecast to surpass half a billion in the UK in 2016.* Mintel Press Report Accessed 29/9/18 at http://www.mintel.com/press-centre/food-and-drink/free-from-gains-momentum-sales-of-free-from-food-products-forecast-to-surpass-half-a-billion-in-the-uk-in-2016 .

Mintel Press Team (2015) *Half of Americans think gluten-free diets are a fad while 25% eat gluten-free foods*. Mintel Press Office Accessed 1/7/18 at http://www.mintel.com/press-centre/food-and-drink/half-of-americans-think-gluten-free-diets-are-a-fad-while-25-eat-gluten-free-foods .

Missbach, B., Schwingshackl, L., Billmann, A., Mystek, A., *et al* (2015). Gluten-free food database: the nutritional quality and cost of packaged gluten-free foods. *PeerJ, 3*, e1337.

Monash University (nd) *What are FODMAPS?* Accessed 11/6/18 at https://www.monashfodmap.com/about-fodmap-and-ibs/.

Mulder, C.J.J.; van Wanrooij, R.L.J.; Bakker, S.F.; Wierdsma, N. and Bouma, G. (2013) Gluten-Free Diet in Gluten-Related Disorders. *Digestive Diseases 31*, 57–62.

Murray, J.A.; Tureka Watson, T.; Clearman, B. and Mitros, F. (2004) Effect of a gluten-free diet on gastrointestinal symptoms in celiac disease. *The American Journal of Clinical Nutrition 79,* 4, 669–673.

NHS UK (2017) *Symptoms: Type 2 Diabetes.* Accessed 3/5/18 at https://www.nhs.uk/conditions/type-2-diabetes/symptoms/.

Offord, C. (2017) *The Celiac Surge* Accessed 1/5/18 at https://www.the-scientist.com/features/the-celiac-surge-31438.

Pulido, O.M; Gillespie, Z.; Zarkadas, M.; Dubois, S.; *et al* (2009) Introduction of oats in the diet of individuals with celiac disease: a systematic review. *Advances in Food and Nutrition Research 57,* 235–85.

Real, A., Comino, I., de Lorenzo L., Mercha, N. F., *et al* (2012) Molecular and Immunological Characterization of Gluten Proteins Isolated from Oat Cultivars That Differ in Toxicity for Celiac Disease. *PLoS ONE 7,* 12.

Reid, J.; Allen, K. and McDonald, S. (2016) *Systematic Review of Safe Level of Gluten for People with Coeliac Disease,* FINAL REPORT 5 February 2016), Cochrane Australia (pdf).

Reilly, N.R. (2016) The Gluten-Free Diet: Recognizing Fact, Fiction, and Fad. *The Journal of Pediatrics 175,* 206-210.

Sapone, A.; Bai, J.C.; Ciacci, C.; Dolinsek, J.; *et al* (2012) Spectrum of gluten-related disorders: Consensus on new nomenclature and classification. *BMC Med. 10*, 13.

Sarwar, M.H.; Sarwar, M.F.; Sarwar M.; Qadri, N.A. and Moghal, S. (2013) The importance of cereals (Poaceae: Gramineae) nutrition in human health: A review. *Journal of Cereals and Oilseeds 4*, 3, 32-35.

Scientific Advisory Committee on Nutrition (2015) *Carbohydrates and Health*. London, TSO.

Shewry, P.R. and Hey, S.J. (2016) Do we need to worry about eating wheat? *Nutrition Bulletin 41*, 6–13.

Silano, M.; Pozo, E.P.; Uberti, F.; Manderfelli, S.; *et al* (2014) Diversity of oat varieties in eliciting the early inflammatory events in celiac disease. European. *Journal of Nutrition 53*, 1177–1186.

Skodje, G.I.; Sarna, V.K.; Minelle, I.H.; Rolfsen, K.L.; *et al* (2017) Fructan, Rather Than Gluten, Induces Symptoms In Patients With Self-reported Non-celiac Gluten Sensitivity. *Gastroenterology 154*, 529-539.

Soares, F.L.P., de Oliveira Matoso, R., Teixeira, L.G., Menezes, Z., *et al* (2013) Gluten-free diet reduces adiposity, inflammation and insulin resistance associated with the induction of PPAR-alpha and PPAR-gamma expression. *Journal of nutritional biochemistry 24*, 105e1111.

Spiller, R. (2017) How do FODMAPS work? *Journal of Gastroenterology and Hepatology 32*, 1, 36–39.

Syage, J.A.; Kelly, C.P.; Dickason, M.A.; Ramirez, A.C.; *et al* (2018) Determination of gluten consumption in celiac disease patients on a gluten-free diet. *American Journal of Clinical Nutrition 107*, 201–207.

The Hartman Group I. *The Hartman Group's Health & Wellness 2015 and Organic & Natural 2014 reports.* http://www.hartman-group.com/acumenPdfs/gluten-free-2015-09-03.pdf.

Threapleton, D. E.; Greenwood, D. C.; Evans, C. E. L.; Cleghorn, C. L.; *et al* (2013) Dietary fibre intake and risk of cardiovascular disease: systematic review and meta-analysis. *British Medical Journal 347*:f6879.

Topper A. (2014) *Non-celiacs Drive Gluten-Free Market Growth.* Mintel Group Ltd. Blog. Accessed 5/5/18 at http://www.mintel.com/blog/food-market-news/gluten-freeconsumption-trends.

Transparency Market Research (2018) *Global Gluten Free Products Market to be Worth S$4.8 bn by 2021-end Growing at a CAGR of 7.70% over 2015-2021.* Accessed 22/8/18 at https://www.transparencymarketresearch.com/pressrelease/gluten-free-products-market.htm.

Valletta, E. and Cipolli, M. (2010) Celiac disease and obesity: Need for nutritional follow-up after diagnosis. *European Journal of Clinical Nutrition, 64*, 1371–1372.

Van Berge-Henegouwen, G.P. and Mulder, C.J. (1993) Pioneer in the gluten free diet: Willem-Karel Dicke 1905–1962, over 50 years of gluten free diet. *Gut 34*, 1473–1475.

van den Broeck, H. C.; Hein C. de Jong, H.C.; Salentijn, E.M.J.; *et al* (2010) Presence of celiac disease epitopes in modern and old hexaploid wheat varieties: wheat breeding may have contributed to increased prevalence of celiac disease. *Theoretical and Applied Genetics 121*, 1527–1539.

Vazquez-Roque, M.I.; Camilleri, M.; Smirk, T.; Murray, J.A.; *et al* (2013) A controlled trial of gluten-free diet in patients with irritable bowel syndrome-diarrhea: Effects on bowel frequency and intestinal function. *Gastroenterology 144*, 903–911.

Verma, A.K.; Gatti, S.; Galeazzi, T.; Monachesi, C.; *et al* (2017) Gluten Contamination in Naturally or Labeled Gluten-Free Products Marketed in Italy, *Nutrients 9*, 115.

Welstead, L. (2015) The Gluten-Free Diet in the 3rd Millennium: Rules, Risks and Opportunities. *Diseases 3*, 3, 136-149.

White, L.E.; Merrick, V.M.; Bannerman, E.; Russell, R.K.; Dharam Basude, D.; Henderson, P.; Wilson , D.C. and Gillett, P.M. (2013) The Rising Incidence of Celiac Disease in Scotland. *Pediatrics 132*; e924.

Williams, P.G. (2012) Evaluation of the evidence between consumption of refined grains and health outcomes. *Nutrition Reviews 20*, 2, 80-99.

World Gastroenterology Organisation (nd) *WGO Practice Guideline - Celiac Disease*. Accessed 1/11/18 at http://www.worldgastroenterology.org/guidelines/global-guidelines/celiac-disease#Ref003.

Wu, J. H. Y., Neal, B., Trevena, H., Crino, M., *et al* (2015). Are gluten-free foods healthier than non-gluten-free foods? An evaluation of supermarket products in Australia. *The British Journal of Nutrition 114*, 3, 448–54.

Ye, E.Q.; Chacko, S.A.; Chou, E.L.; Kugizaki, M. and Liu, S. (2012) Greater whole-grain intake is associated with lower risk of type 2 diabetes, cardiovascular disease, and weight gain. *The Journal of Nutrition 142*, 1304-13.

Zong, G.; Lebwohl, B.; Frank Hu, F.; Sampson, L.; *et al* (2017) Abstract 11: Associations of Gluten Intake With Type 2 Diabetes Risk and Weight Gain in Three Large Prospective Cohort Studies of US Men and Women. *Circulation 135*, A11.